THE
COUPLES'
PREGNANCY
GUIDE

THE COUPLES' PREGNANCY GUIDE

How to Navigate Pregnancy
and Childbirth as a Team

D'ANTHONY & RACHEL WARD

ZEITGEIST · NEW YORK

Published in the United States by Zeitgeist, an imprint of Zeitgeist™, a division of Penguin Random House LLC, New York.

penguinrandomhouse.com

Zeitgeist™ is a trademark of Penguin Random House LLC

ISBN: 9780593436059
Ebook ISBN: 9780593436042

Author photograph © by André Brown of André Brown Photography
Cover design by Nami Kurita
Interior design by Emma Hall
Edited by Clara Song Lee

Printed in the United States of America
1 3 5 7 9 10 8 6 4 2

First Edition

To our children, Taj and Aaliyah.

You are an amazing inspiration for growth

and maturity for us. It is because of you that

we can share this book with the world.

We love you!

CONTENTS

INTRODUCTION

As we sit in our living room, Rachel feeding Aaliyah and D'Anthony playing with Taj, we can't help but reminisce about the two pregnancy journeys that have brought us here. Beautiful, educational, and eventful journeys filled with excitement from month to month as we anxiously awaited—and then experienced—all the pregnancy milestones we had only heard about. And now we are so excited to help you begin your first pregnancy journey together!

But first, a little bit about ourselves: We are D'Anthony and Rachel Ward, partners in life and parents of two beautiful children, Taj and Aaliyah. We're a Black millennial couple whose world lit up with a new understanding of "family" when we became parents—so much so that becoming a father inspired D'Anthony to launch *The Dad Vlog*, a digital-content brand that celebrates the simple joys of raising a family. Now, together, we're excited to join forces to share with you our story as a couple, as you begin your own momentous journey through pregnancy, childbirth, and life with your own unique and miraculous creation.

What's special about this book is that it's as much focused on you two as a couple as it is on pregnancy or parenting. It's about how to navigate the various stages and challenges you will inevitably face together with grace and efficiency, and with a commitment to teamwork with the precious person you've chosen to take this life walk with. It's about making your parenting story work for you, because these defining times will teach you so much about each other; hopefully enough that you feel, going forward, you can conquer anything as a team.

But so much of life isn't big challenges. Much of life involves every-dayness, the potentially mundane. And it's easy to let these moments fly by without notice. When we were pregnant with our eldest, Taj, we often found ourselves jumping ahead, debating on which HBCU he would attend, or what gift we would get him for his 16th birthday. By the time we were pregnant with Aaliyah, we'd gotten more adept at appreciating all the little everyday details. Throughout all this, we knew there would be many moments, and many decisions to be made. And instead of agonizing over every little decision, we took comfort in knowing that any decision that was made, we made it together.

THE KEY TO SUCCESS

Most days, we feel like a well-oiled machine; we divide and conquer as needed and complete each other's unfinished tasks without much prompting. Routines make it easy to know who takes care of what: If D'Anthony gives Taj his bath, Rachel gets Aaliyah ready for bed. We pay attention to what's happening for the other person so we can help out if needed. Life is still chaotic—we're working parents with two small children, after all—but we appreciate every day, and our marriage feels as strong as ever.

But it wasn't always this way. During our first pregnancy, D'Anthony felt very strongly that Rachel needed to stay as stress-free as possible, focusing solely on taking care of herself and the growing baby and leaving him to take care of everything else, including her half of our two-person household. But as the weeks passed, we quickly realized that this wasn't realistic—nine months of this would've taken a major toll on D'Anthony and worn him out before the baby even arrived—so we adjusted our approach.

We discovered that teamwork is 85 percent mental and emotional; we need to tune in to each other and respond accordingly, or else things just don't go smoothly. With that realization, we chose a new approach—to take care of each other while sharing the load in ways that felt right for each of us. Throughout, we learned to communicate better, to do check-ins with each other and get on the same page, even when things got stressful and tiring.

There is no right or wrong when it comes to teamwork in your pregnancy journey—everyone's experiences will be unique and different. But the ability to sense each other's needs and respond or adjust accordingly—what relationship experts call "emotional attunement"—is foundational to our success as partners and as parents. When you're attuned to each other, life's challenges—be they intense pregnancy side effects or middle-of-the-night feedings with a newborn—feel a lot less intimidating because you know you're not alone: You're navigating them *together*.

HOW TO USE THIS BOOK

When we set out to write this book, our goal wasn't to provide scientific or medical advice on pregnancy. That's not us—trust in your healthcare professionals to help with that. Instead, we wanted to fulfill a need that we've seen within our community of first-time parents, to answer the question *What the heck are we getting ourselves into, and how do we get through this together?* How could we help first-time parents get a better sense of all the things they need to look into so they can channel their pregnancy-inspired energy in useful ways? And be a strong team doing so?

The result is a collection of practical advice, tools, and checklists that can help you figure out what you need to address and plan for in the next nine months and beyond. Because everyone's pregnancy journey is different, some of what we share may not apply to you. Just take what resonates and leave behind anything that doesn't suit your family and situation.

The chapters are organized in time order, based on the baby's growth. Each chapter opens with brief descriptions of the physical changes happening for the baby and the pregnant partner, as well as

Team Toolbox sections, in which we provide tips and strategies that have worked for us in the corresponding months. Considerations and Expectations sections cover topics that are worth looking into and important decisions that may need to be made that month. Divide and Conquer checklists help couples share responsibilities or divvy up tasks and Decide Together worksheets provide guidance for brainstorming solutions together when you face tricky decisions. Chapter sidebars offer additional discussions for subjects that deserve more attention, like what to do when finances feel tight, how to keep intimacy alive, or why it's so important to advocate for yourselves in medical settings. For glimpses into Rachel's or D'Anthony's individual perspectives, check out the In Her Words and In His Words boxes sprinkled throughout. Finally, if you need additional space to jot down your thoughts, you'll find blank pages for notes at the end of the book.

PART ONE

———

THE
FIRST
TRIMESTER

From Period to Pregnant

"I'm late! I need to take a pregnancy test!"

"I'm ovulating, let's go for it!"

Which one was it for you? Between our pregnancies with Taj and Aaliyah, we have experienced both the "Wait, what?" and the "Let's try." Regardless of how you got here, you are here. Congratulations! Try to use this month to enjoy each other and take in the moment.

WHAT'S PHYSICALLY HAPPENING

Calling it the first month of pregnancy is a tad misleading because, technically, people aren't actually pregnant until the middle of it. Week 1 is counted from the first day of the pregnant person's last menstrual cycle, and doctors use this timing (known as gestational age) to track your pregnancy and the baby's development. In a typical cycle, conception doesn't happen until around week 3, after ovulation occurs and the sperm fertilizes the egg. By the end of week 4, your future baby has set up shop in the uterine lining and settled in for the long haul. Based on this timing, the baby will actually develop for 38 weeks (full-term pregnancy), even though the pregnancy count started two weeks earlier.

In terms of symptoms, it's common for a lot of people to not notice this first month, since their first sign of pregnancy is a missed period. For us, we didn't realize we were pregnant with Taj until week 5 when Rachel missed her period. This was true again for our pregnancy with Aaliyah, even though we were actively tracking Rachel's cycle and trying to get pregnant. For that pregnancy, we took a pregnancy test three weeks after ovulation and discovered Rachel was pregnant again at week 5. So we missed month one for both of our pregnancies!

TEAM TOOLBOX

This Month's Strategy: Emo Deposits

Pregnancy is a life-changing experience, and everything changes again when a baby enters the picture. Our first piece of advice for preparing emotionally and mentally as a team: Get in the habit of showing how much you care for and appreciate each other. We don't mean the occasional "thanks" here and there. Relationship experts contend that when couples build up a cushion of intentional, positive interactions, it can make tough times easier to get through. Research also shows that focusing on small, positive things every day strengthens relationships better than the occasional grand gesture.

In our case, we try to make "emo deposits" in each other's "love accounts." The "emo" is short for "emotional" and refers to thoughtful gestures we do to show emotional support. For example, when we found out Rachel was pregnant with our son, Taj, D'Anthony went on YouTube and found weekly videos of a typical baby's development inside the belly. The videos were incredibly cheesy, but we had four weeks of information to catch up on, and Rachel appreciated D'Anthony's enthusiasm and interest. It can also refer to physical actions we take to show we care, such as giving a foot rub without being asked or running to the store to pick up a favorite snack.

You'll find your own ways of making emo deposits, but the idea is to make intentional effort to let your partner know that you love them, notice what they're doing, and appreciate the things they do for you and your family.

A few more things to note with emo deposits:

FREQUENCY MATTERS. Consistent small gestures are better than occasional big gestures (though big gestures are always appreciated).

NO GESTURE IS TOO SMALL. A quick compliment, giving a back hug while your partner washes the dishes, offering your partner the last cookie—it all counts.

EXPRESS GRATITUDE. When you notice receiving an emo deposit, let your partner know you appreciate it!

In the first month of pregnancy, emo deposits can go a long way in reassuring each other that you're all in, no matter how you feel about what's happening around you. If you're the non-birthing partner, doing things like researching hospitals and childbirth classes or giving an extra hug or two throughout the day lets an anxious pregnant person know that you plan to be present and engaged throughout the process.

And if you're the pregnant person, asking your partner about their feelings and letting them express their joys or concerns without judgment shows you trust them and want to make space for their experience, too. After all, you're in this together!

CONSIDERATIONS AND EXPECTATIONS

You may not know what to expect, and it's not uncommon among first-time parents to feel a swirl of emotions. Or a tsunami. There are two pieces of advice that can help prepare you mentally and emotionally for the pregnancy experience.

1. DON'T PANIC ABOUT THE PAST.

If you are the pregnant partner, it's normal to have moments of concern about what you ate, drank, or did in the past that could potentially affect your pregnancy. An internet search will provide a list of one million "things you shouldn't do while pregnant." And of those things, you may have done half already. What's done is done, so there's no point in panicking. It's better for you and your baby if you commit to making thoughtful choices starting now—this is a great time to make lifestyle changes that will help you and your baby thrive going forward.

As the non-birthing partner, you can help by reassuring your pregnant partner that the obstetrician or other healthcare provider will answer all their questions and concerns at your first appointment. The sooner you both learn to set healthy boundaries with what random strangers on the internet say, the easier your lives will be. This is applicable not just for pregnancy but for your parenting journey, too. (Oh, and life in general!)

2. APPRECIATE EVERY DAY.

This point might seem trite, but we believe it's important to notice the day-to-day moments that weave together and form the fabric of life. Whether you call it mindfulness or living in the present moment, for us, slowing down and being intentional about noticing everyday moments has made a huge difference in our sense of well-being and happiness. Researchers say this is because when you practice gratitude, you create a habit of looking for new things to be grateful about. That generates a cycle in which you feel grateful more often, which inspires you to look for more things to be grateful for, and the feelings of gratitude just amplify and grow.

After doing this gratitude thing for a while, our mindset shifted to one that genuinely appreciates everything about our lives, from the major blessings (we love you, Taj and Aaliyah!) to the everyday little moments, like the way Taj cracks himself up over silly jokes that make sense only to him, and the radiant smile Aaliyah gives us when we enter her room after her nap. When you realize and take note of the good things in your overall life, the tough things feel a little less intense.

This month, while there isn't a whole lot you *have* to do, shifting your perspective, either by ramping up the emo deposits or practicing gratitude daily, can make a huge difference for your overall pregnancy journey. Whatever your circumstances, we hope you'll find a perspective that brings more empathy, appreciation, and peace into your life.

Taking the Test

It's recommended to consult with an obstetric provider at about 8 weeks, so you can start looking into finding one (see page 32 for more on this). In the meantime, let's talk about the only thing you may want to do this month: take a pregnancy test.

Note that most health savings accounts and flexible spending accounts cover the cost of pregnancy tests. Home pregnancy tests are up to 99 percent accurate, as long as you use them correctly and wait until the first day of your expected period.

When you're ready to take the test, try to make it fun and reduce any anxiety. If you're excited about getting pregnant, you can document the moment with pictures and videos. If you haven't discussed pregnancy together a whole lot, try not to make any assumptions about how you'll both feel. It's a big moment, and you may be surprised to discover that one of you will need more support than the other.

We highly recommend testing together. It's a great foundational start to this journey to find out the results together. Whether you get a positive or negative test result, or a happy or sad response, they are all valid, and it's okay to take some time to absorb the results. With our first (unexpected) pregnancy, Rachel's initial response included a few choice words and the need to take some time for herself. By the time she came out of her state of shock, though, D'Anthony was right there to offer support.

We also recommend taking the test on a day when you don't have any other commitments. This will allow both of you time to process in the way you feel most comfortable for as long as you need, without feeling rushed. It also allows for some spontaneous celebration if you choose.

After the Test

Once you've gotten a positive test, pick up some prenatal vitamins (make sure it includes folate or folic acid) to kick-start healthy development for baby *and* mom. Then take some time to savor the news, just between the two of you. Resist the urge to jump into the deep end—there will be plenty of time to talk about finding a doctor, picking a name, revealing the sex, deciding where to live, etc. All of that is coming, so today, enjoy the moment.

If you're ready to celebrate, do so! Go out for a fancy dinner, have a romantic night in, take a spontaneous road trip; do whatever excites the two of you. And since you're pretty much two seconds pregnant, it's okay to ease into a healthy pregnant lifestyle. This doesn't mean you should run out and do shots at a bar, but nor do you want to immediately stress yourself out trying to pick out the healthiest meal on the menu or quit your morning cup of coffee cold turkey, either. Learning to balance your mental stress levels with the physical needs of the baby will be an ongoing practice, so be gentle as you both adjust to your new stage of life—as a pregnant couple!

In His Words

While we were dating, I asked Rachel if she would be okay if we got pregnant. Her answer was "Yeah, I'd be fine if that were to happen." Fast-forward to the day we found out she was pregnant. Complete and utter shock. I had to give her time to process and go through the ups and downs that come with such a life-changing experience. You never truly know how you'll feel about something—especially something major like pregnancy—until you're in the moment (and even after the moment)!

Fertility Struggles, Pregnancy Loss, and Difficult News

Every pregnancy is different. People with eight kids will tell you in great detail how their eight pregnancies differed wildly. That said, no pregnancy journey is perfect, and they each come with unique challenges. Unfortunately, some are much harder than others, sometimes even before they begin.

Fertility issues can result in yearslong struggles to conceive and an accompanying roller coaster of emotions. And miscarriages are heartbreaking to endure, the loss of a life and all the dreams of what might have been. But there is comfort in knowing that you are not alone if you have dealt with either of these difficult experiences. Things like fertility struggles and miscarriages are far more common than people often realize, and there are many support systems available (see Resources, page 172).

Regardless of your unique experience with loss, the aftermath is often really hard for couples, who may process feelings differently. Our friends Amy and Anthony, whose baby was stillborn, reflected: "It's hard to cope with. We should have gotten a therapist to help us through it. We were detached."

There is no manual for coping with a pregnancy struggle or loss, and there is no right or wrong way to deal with it. Listening to our friends' story, it was clear that they fully leaned on each other for support, which is ultimately what got them through their grief. Their experience, though tragic, also led to a transformation in their relationship that brought them closer together and solidified their bond.

DIVIDE AND CONQUER

For each month, we'll provide a simple to-do list to get you thinking about tasks or research that may be pertinent this month or in preparation for upcoming months. This isn't a comprehensive list or a rule book—it just provides some general direction, so take what you need, leave what you don't, and simply use our advice as a possible starting point for your own research.

For non-birthing partners, as you review these lists each month, take some time to assess how your pregnant partner is feeling, mentally and physically, and how much they may be able to take on for that month. See where you can pick up some of the slack. Over time, the way you divvy up work may shift and change, especially as your partner's fatigue and physical discomfort ebb and flow.

For the first month, remember that the focus is wrapping your head around this whole new stage, and hopefully it's fun and low-stress. We've intentionally kept this month's list short with just a couple of key items to get you grounded in your new reality and prepared for next month.

TIME-SENSITIVE

- Pregnancy test
- Prenatal vitamins

SCHEDULE AND PLAN

- Time to enjoy each other's company

RESEARCH AND DISCUSS

- Remedies for pregnancy side effects like morning sickness
- Choosing a healthcare provider (page 32)

ADDITIONAL

_____

_____

_____

_____

_____

DECIDE TOGETHER

Use these sheets to help you get on the same page when you're facing a tricky decision, like choosing a name or figuring out childcare.

YOUR PROBLEM OR DESIRED GOAL: _____

_____

What's important to Partner A?	What's important to Partner B?

Circle the top one to three things that matter most to you. Take turns explaining to your partner why your circled items are important to you. Then take some time separately to research and brainstorm solutions. List all your ideas, even wild or unusual ones.

_____

_____

_____

_____

_____

_____

_____

List any factors that will impact your decision. This is where you set reasonable boundaries (time, cost, effort, etc.) about your possible solutions.

_____

_____

_____

_____

_____

_____

_____

_____

_____

Partner A's short list	Partner B's short list

Discuss which solution is best for your relationship. Can you come to an enthusiastic agreement?

OUR FINAL DECISION: _____

Taking Stock

Ready to make things happen? This month, the pregnancy seems a bit more real with some added responsibilities. There will likely be googling, doctor office visits, and more, and there may be a little nausea with some fatigue. You and your partner may feel immense elation, or nervousness and fearfulness. Either way, it's normal and we see you, and there are things you can do as your pregnancy moves forward to champion your cause and feel more in control.

WHAT'S PHYSICALLY HAPPENING

One of the most fun aspects of pregnancy is tracking the growth of your baby. We made this part even more interesting and intimate by sitting down together every Sunday night and watching a weekly video on baby development. It highlighted all the changes the baby was going through as they developed. We really enjoyed these videos because they filled the learning gap between doctor visits. Check out Resources (page 172) for the weekly video series we watched.

In this book, we've compared the size of the baby with different fruits and vegetables. For month two, a commonly used comparison is a raspberry. At this point, your baby has a brain and their limbs are starting to grow. You'll likely get your first ultrasound this month, where you will probably see that your baby's head is far larger than the rest of their body—you'll also get the chance to hear your baby's heartbeat for the first time!

Now on to the maybe-not-so-fun part: Increased hormones may cause mood swings and nausea. Not all pregnant people will experience the infamous "morning sickness," but for those who do, it will likely start this month. The experience of morning sickness will vary from person to person; even our experience between the first and second pregnancy was very different.

In Her Words

Imagine being at "the Most Magical Place on Earth," celebrating your birthday on a surprise trip. There's Mickey, frolicking gleefully through the streets, and a smile on every face you see—but you are locked in the bathroom, hot, nauseous, and crying. That was me two months pregnant with Taj. Alternately, imagine closing on your first home and you're at the bank trying to wire the down payment needed to finish the transaction, but you run out of the bank manager's office to vomit in the bushes next to a stranger using the ATM. That was also me, pregnant at two months with Aaliyah. I wish you a much different experience!

Nausea or vomiting during pregnancy is called morning sickness because it usually happens in the morning. But it can last all day long. Hopefully, you'll escape this phase unscathed. But if you find nausea is an issue, here are a few helpful tips:

EAT FIRST THING IN THE MORNING. You can even keep crackers on your nightstand.

EAT FREQUENT SMALL MEALS. Don't wait until hunger hits. Carry snacks with you at all times.

STAY HYDRATED. Making a human requires a lot of water, so double your intake. Make it a habit to carry a water bottle.

TRY PROTEIN SHAKES. In cases of vomiting or difficulty eating, protein shakes are a quick and easy way to get some nutrients down.

HOLD OFF ON TRIPS OR LONG DRIVES. Focus on adjusting to your pregnancy. You can always plan to take trips in later months.

RESEARCH HOME REMEDIES. We found ginger tea helpful for settling a queasy stomach.

ASK YOUR HEALTHCARE PROVIDER. Keep your provider up to date on symptoms, as sometimes there are prescription medication options that can help.

Non-birthing person, you may feel helpless, but there are plenty of heroic deeds available to you. You can provide backup support, such as offering a wet washcloth for your partner's forehead, or taking over whatever task they dropped to tend to their nausea. Bring your own stash of crackers and a water bottle so you can jump in and offer them when your partner suddenly feels nauseous, weak, or hangry.

TEAM TOOLBOX

This Month's Strategy: Check-Ins

"Soo . . . how do you feel about all this?" D'Anthony questioned Rachel when we discovered we were pregnant with Taj.

"You're obviously excited," she replied.

This kind of questioning was D'Anthony's way of starting our check-ins. Check-ins are regular talks that allow us to chat through how we're feeling and anything that's coming up for us in our relationship.

This month, we'll share our strategies for check-ins, so you can intentionally lean on each other for support and take specific actions to gauge how your partner is feeling. We learned early on in our marriage that the old cliché that "communication is key" actually *is* key.

How to check in:

1. First, set the environment for these check-ins. Make sure you're dedicating your undivided attention to these moments. Set aside at least half an hour of quiet time. If the TV is on, shut it off. Set your phone aside. And if you're cooking, wait until it's time to eat. For many couples, it helps to schedule recurring check-ins on their calendar.

2. Once the mood is set, start the check-in the same way each time. In our case, we knew a check-in was starting when one of us said "Let's talk" or "Soooo . . ." while sitting in the living room, chatting over dinner, or going for a walk. You can make it as romantic or casual as you like. Some couples might light a candle in preparation, open with a long hug, or gaze into each other's eyes before talking. Others might prefer to make it more fun, like by setting out drinks and snacks.

3. Get chatting and listening. The goal is to talk openly about what's going on for each other and share anything that feels pressing or worthy of some attention. Ideally, you'll each have the chance to

talk about your feelings uninterrupted, without implying blame or getting defensive.

4. End the check-in on a high note, perhaps by talking about some wins you've had as a couple and expressing gratitude to each other.

If you're stumped on how to start, the following questions might generate some good check-ins. Just pick one or two per check-in—no need to go through this entire list! Make sure each partner gets a turn to respond:

- What went well for us this week? What didn't go so well, and how can we fix it?

- How did I make you feel loved this week? Is there anything I can do more regularly to make you feel loved and appreciated?

- Is there something I did that upset you? How can I make it better?

- Is there anything stressing you out these days? How can I help?

- Is there anything else you want to share with me?

You may ask your partner a question, and they may express a thought that differs from your feelings on the matter. If that's the case, knowing this can help you support each other better. With regard to pregnancy, you may have very different views at first. It's also common to have a delayed or evolving response to the thought of having a baby. Initially it may start off as excitement, then as the days go by, perhaps excitement is replaced by shock or fear, or vice versa. Whatever the response, give each other the permission to experience these different emotions.

CONSIDERATIONS AND EXPECTATIONS

If you're the pregnant person, you may have started to experience some of the physical challenges previously discussed. You'll also want to find a healthcare provider and get on board with regular appointments. At the same time, you'll both begin to figure out what expenses you can expect in the coming months. As the momentum builds, we'll explore how to manage the loads—mental and physical—between you and your partner.

Your Medical Provider(s)

Finding the right OB-GYN (obstetrician-gynecologist) will set the foundation for your medical guidance throughout the entire pregnancy. We didn't have an OB-GYN when we got pregnant with Taj, and we relocated shortly after getting pregnant with Aaliyah, so we had to go through the search process twice. Both times, we started with friends' recommendations and a search through our insurance provider. For us, it was important to have a seasoned doctor who looked like us and wasn't too far from where we lived, which led to internet searches and hospital websites to find photos and biographies and read reviews. A family member also helped by calling some OB-GYN offices and asking the nurses and staff their opinion of the doctor. People are surprisingly honest! Also, feel free to meet with a couple of OB-GYNs before making a final decision.

We believe that one of the most important aspects of selecting an OB-GYN is bedside manner. Ask yourself, *How responsive and patient is the doctor with our concerns/questions? How clearly do they explain information? How much time did they spend with us?* The bottom line is, do you feel heard, cared for, and comfortable with this person?

At your first appointment, you may see a midwife, physician's assistant, or nurse practitioner instead of the OB-GYN to confirm your pregnancy and discuss their practice and what to expect from your healthcare throughout the pregnancy timeline. Before this first meeting, put together a list of any questions you may have about the practice and doctor to see if they are a good fit. Include questions about your pregnancy to get information on what diet and lifestyle changes they recommend. Most OB-GYN offices will provide a list of allowed medications while pregnant and a list of foods that are no longer safe to eat. Non-birthing partners, listen in to the guidance around diet and lifestyle so you can support them in making positive choices. If you want, you can join them in living a healthier lifestyle so you create a sense of solidarity. Building good habits now will help throughout the pregnancy and after the baby comes, when things get busier!

Logistics and Finances

In a few short months, your home will be filled with the sights and sounds of a brand-new person! It's easy to get caught up in visions of how this will feel and look, but it's equally important to map out the logistics. When you walk through your home, ask yourself: *Where will baby sleep? What is our proximity to the baby? Do we have pets to consider? Is the home ready and safe; that is, do we need to address any concerns?* It's never too early to start talking through how things may look.

More important, now is a good time to start talking about finances. Not always a fun discussion, but an important one. It's no surprise that there is a tremendous financial responsibility that comes along with a child. The most surprising aspect for us was the cost of the actual pregnancy. Since everyone's financial situation is different, there is no one-size-fits-all in approaching the financial responsibility. But planning and research can go a long way.

Talk to an adviser if you like, or just sit down together and hash it out a bit. Are there cost-cutting measures you can take to reprioritize where your money goes? For families who qualify, this is an excellent time to look into state-funded or federally funded programs that can assist with specific needs such as healthcare, housing, food, etc. (More on financial strategies on page 80.)

With both Taj and Aaliyah, we took advantage of the benefits of a health savings account (HSA). An HSA allows you to save money tax-free and use it toward medical costs like doctor appointments and prescriptions. And here's where you can really benefit: Whatever your annual deductible is, try to work together to deposit that amount into the HSA. It may take four or five months, but your deductible will be tax-free, and you will reach your deductible with the cost of the birth alone. If you're planning your pregnancy and the timing of your benefits enrollment aligns with your plans, then you may want to select the highest coverage plan for the year you plan to give birth.

Here are some additional costs you'll want to consider:

CHILDCARE. Start to think about your childcare options, if needed, and whether one of you will be a stay-at-home parent. Is it realistic to have a family member or friend help (be sure to ask; don't assume!), or will you need to select a day care for your child? Childcare is by far our largest monthly bill, next to our mortgage. Depending on where you live, you can expect monthly childcare costs averaging $1,230.

PARENTAL LEAVE. Depending on your work situation, you may be able to take parental leave after the baby arrives. Some companies offer fully paid parental leave while other employers will not be able to offer any paid benefits. You'll want to discuss strategies for bridging the gap during this time, whether through cost-cutting measures and/or increased saving during the pregnancy months. One option for couples where both partners work: Stagger the parental leaves so there is more coverage before the baby enters childcare. For both children, D'Anthony split his parental leave into two periods, one short period used right after the birth, and the remainder used once Rachel returned to work.

PREGNANCY AND DELIVERY BILLS. If someone gives you an aspirin at the hospital, you can expect to get a bill for it! There are lots of folks on the ground and behind the scenes when a baby is born and in the months leading up to it. Two strategies for minimizing the costs: (1) Ensure that your providers, including the birth anesthesiologist, are in your insurance company's network; (2) Negotiate payment plans, and if a surprise bill comes along, make payments (even small ones) as regularly as possible.

FINANCIAL ACCOUNTS. It's never too early to start saving for college! If regular deposits into an account aren't in your budget right now, no worries. Keep it in mind for the future, though, and in the meantime, start small. Coins in a water jug add up, too.

How (and When) to Share the News

One last item to consider is when and how to share the pregnancy news with family and friends. Some couples want to share from the moment they find out, and some want to wait until the first trimester is over because the chances of miscarriage drop significantly at that point. There is no "right" answer except "when you are both comfortable."

With both pregnancies, we waited until we saw our family in person, specifically our parents, since we lived in a different state from the majority of our family. We used those visits to share the news—with Taj, at four months, and with Aaliyah, two months. For siblings and other close family members and friends, Taj's announcement came in the form of a story line within a photo booth strip that we mailed to family and friends. Aaliyah's announcement was a picture of Taj wearing a "Big Brother" shirt that we sent out by text.

Pregnancy announcements can be as simple as a phone call or as involved as a professional photo shoot. If you don't plan to do a gender-reveal party, you could do a pregnancy-reveal party instead. Don't get hung up on the "how"; just do whatever feels natural. The one caveat: If you have a beloved aunt who doesn't "do" social media, give her a call to share the news—it's never good to face the repercussions of a close family member who hears the big news through the grapevine!

Sharing the Mental Load

It's no secret that historically, women and birthing people have been asked to juggle a lot—taking care of a household, raising a family, and engaging in paid work come to mind, just for starters. As a result, it seems like they've developed this incredible ability to store dozens of things in their brain, like an extensive to-do list. But mixed in with this may be some thoughts and feelings that they want to say out loud but have been conditioned to not do so. Add things like pregnancy, appointments, and nausea, and this "mental load" can increase exponentially. As the non-birthing partner, you can help relieve the pressure that is historically placed on women and pregnant people by proactively taking care of tasks and "owning" more responsibilities—without waiting to be asked to help. There is nothing more pleasurable to a nauseous pregnant person than hearing the words "I already took care of it."

In our case, Rachel often would think about things that needed to be completed at home, her performance at work, or managing things for her parents and family. It became more apparent to D'Anthony that she needed more support during her pregnancies. The problem was, it was impossible for him to understand everything that was going through her head, and Rachel didn't always have the time or energy to explicitly lay out all the things she felt she needed to do. Nor did she want to keep asking him to help her.

To make things easier, D'Anthony began paying more attention to things that he knew Rachel did regularly, like washing the dishes before bed or switching the clothes from the washer to the dryer. And—this is key—he began taking care of these tasks without her asking. When she got out of bed and started to walk toward the kitchen, D'Anthony would say something like, "Where you going?" and she would say, "To do the dishes." He'd respond, "Oh, I did the dishes already." Her body language said more than her words, and her sense of relief was satisfying to him. Over time, it became easier to divvy up more responsibilities and sharing more of the mental load.

Within D'Anthony's circle of male friends, they take on more house-hold responsibilities than we believe studies or statistics would show, and this is as it should be. Some tips on how to make it work:

- Divide responsibilities according to your preferences. Some people loathe doing laundry but don't mind washing dishes. Other people might not mind doing laundry but have a real issue with cleaning bathrooms. Give each other the tasks that you don't mind doing, and take turns handling tasks that you both dislike.

- Go with what's most efficient and aligns with your skill sets. In our family, Rachel takes care of monthly expenses because she's great at staying on top of paperwork, while D'Anthony is in charge of taking photos and videos of the family because that's part of his day job.

- Try to divide work in a way that feels right for each of you. If one partner does most of the cooking, can the other partner handle cleanup and grocery shopping? The goal isn't necessarily to divide the work fifty-fifty (that may not be possible, depending on the other responsibilities you each have) but rather to divide the mental load in a way that feels best to each of you.

In the beginning, sharing the mental load will require the pregnant person to vocalize their needs. If you're the non-birthing partner, you may need to remind them to share their thoughts when they're feeling stressed and overwhelmed. But over time, as you continue to get attuned to each other's needs, it will get easier to anticipate what you each need and help each other without needing to be asked.

DIVIDE AND CONQUER

There's plenty for the pregnant partner to do this month, but it's also a perfect time for non-birthing partners to make emo deposits that instill confidence in their partner. Last month, you invested in their confidence by making small, loving gestures. This month, your partner will begin to feel some physical effects of the pregnancy and have additional responsibilities with doctor visits and various appointments. They may be nauseous, and they may have mood swings or be irritable. Look for opportunities to support and take on additional tasks. What you can do is, well, everything you can! If they have a headache, you can grab them a drink of water or acetaminophen, if the doc says it's okay. If they are feeling nauseous, have them sit down and provide a cold, damp compress. These responses may not always end in relief, but they'll know you care. And that's what really counts.

Another way to share the workload is around appointments and load management. To make scheduling easier, share your work calendars with each other so that whoever is making an appointment can do so without having to consult the other person. The pregnant partner may want to take the lead on finding an OB-GYN, but there's no reason not to do this together, since you both can and should engage with the doctor regularly. After an initial visit to confirm the pregnancy, there will be additional checkups at regular intervals to make sure everything is progressing smoothly. There may be separate appointments for blood tests, ultrasounds, and more.

It can be very easy for non-birthing partners to take a back seat approach to this, but there's so much you can do to help. Begin by doing some research before the appointments. This shows your partner that you're interested and engaged, and by researching and gathering important questions to ask at the appointments, you may uncover things that your partner hasn't thought of. If possible, try to attend as many appointments as you can. This shows emotional support, but more important, it allows you to hear the same information that your pregnant partner hears. This can be super helpful later, should your partner become overwhelmed at any point or have trouble following through on all the doctor's guidance.

In His Words

Rachel's pregnancy with Aaliyah was right after the start of the pandemic. Hospitals were not allowing anyone to accompany the patient to their doctor appointments, so I sat in the parking lot and used video chat to ask whatever questions I had. That was a great emo deposit to show Rachel I was all in, no matter the circumstances.

TIME-SENSITIVE

- Find an OB-GYN or midwife
- Schedule first prenatal appointment
- Brainstorm questions for prenatal appointment

SCHEDULE AND PLAN

- When to share pregnancy news
- Baby journal to document your journey
- Couple check-in

RESEARCH AND DISCUSS

- Medical provider options: OB-GYN, midwife, doula (see page 64)
- Guidelines for healthy pregnancy: sleep, diet, exercise, chemical exposure, etc.
- Insurance coverage for family planning, pregnancy, and postpartum care
- Strategies for good sleep
- Weekly baby development video (see Resources, page 172)

ADDITIONAL

- _____
- _____
- _____
- _____
- _____
- _____
- _____

DECIDE TOGETHER

Use these sheets to help you get on the same page when you're facing a tricky decision, like choosing a name or figuring out childcare.

YOUR PROBLEM OR DESIRED GOAL: _____

_____

What's important to Partner A?	What's important to Partner B?

Circle the top one to three things that matter most to you. Take turns explaining to your partner why your circled items are important to you. Then take some time separately to research and brainstorm solutions. List all your ideas, even wild or unusual ones.

_____

_____

_____

_____

_____

_____

List any factors that will impact your decision. This is where you set reasonable boundaries (time, cost, effort, etc.) about your possible solutions.

_____

_____

_____

_____

_____

_____

_____

_____

_____

Partner A's short list	Partner B's short list

Discuss which solution is best for your relationship. Can you come to an enthusiastic agreement?

OUR FINAL DECISION: _____

Adjusting to Changes

It seemed like the world's best-kept secret as we left work early to attend a doctor appointment or politely declined sushi dates with friends or cleverly evaded a glass of wine offered to us. This was our new normal, along with Rachel battling morning sickness while D'Anthony ended up on the eighth page of a Google search looking for nausea-relief strategies. Month three is all about identifying your new normal, becoming accustomed to the changes that are happening, and, most important, positioning your relationship for success.

WHAT'S PHYSICALLY HAPPENING

This is an exciting month in baby development. All the organs and limbs are formed, and now your baby can poop! Baby's size will grow exponentially this month—from the size of a grape to that of a lime.

Nausea may still be an issue. Baby is growing, and so is the uterus, so the pregnant partner may notice a little change in their weight or the way clothes fit. Hopefully it's possible to get a good variety of food down; a prenatal vitamin can help supplement what's not being met.

In Her Words

While three months pregnant with Taj, I went on my annual family vacation to Vegas. I ate breakfast every morning, kept snacks in my room, and got water shots at the bar while everyone else got tequila. I toured casinos and walked the Strip, though I skipped 4D rides because 3D glasses made me nauseous. With Aaliyah, we had just closed on a new home. Because I was so nauseous, I couldn't unpack, and I lost weight due to constant vomiting, which landed me in the ER, dehydrated and needing IV fluids. I was working full-time and had not yet shared the news with my workplace, so I was exhausted. Two pregnancies, two very different experiences.

Excessive stress can be a contributing cause of complications during pregnancy. Non-birthing partners, you can help by taking steps to keep your partner's stress levels down. Great ways to help reduce stress include active listening, finding ways to help, and encouraging relaxation (for both of you!). You might buy your partner a journal that they can vent to, or seek out some mindfulness and meditation videos or apps to enjoy together.

TEAM TOOLBOX

This Month's Strategy: Team Values

Wrapping your head around this new journey requires a level of vulnerability and soul-searching that is incredibly intentional. Depending on where you are in life and the circumstances under which the pregnancy occurred, identifying the values that apply to you both could be a walk in the park or extremely challenging. It's important to identify your values as a team because your shared and collective morals and values will help guide you through the issues that arise. By having a handle on these values, couples can resolve conflicts when they arise and experience effective communication.

Ideally, we never stop growing, and our values may shift and grow throughout our life experience, especially in a shared relationship. For us, we wanted to identify values that could guide us, both during the pregnancy as well as beyond the pregnancy stage. You may feel the need to share the same values; just keep in mind that you each have different needs, and things that will stand out differently to each of you as important. The goal is to find your *shared* values, for these values will be the foundation of your family. You can also work to honor the values that each partner carries independently—these matter, too.

One value that resonated with us during this process was empathy. Empathy is the ability to understand and share feelings with each other, and it plays an especially big role during pregnancy. You can imagine how this is important from both perspectives. The pregnant person is going through an unprecedented body and life change, and their thought process is focused on coping with all the change. The ability to understand this will help the pregnancy go much more smoothly and safely, as they will be less stressed, and the non-birthing partner will be able to take a step back and acknowledge any changes in behavior. These values are a two-way street: It's equally important for the non-birthing partner to receive empathy as well, with recognition of both their stake in this journey and the life changes and thoughts taking place for them too.

Other values that are important to us are respect, autonomy, and trust. While empathy helps us better understand each other, respect guides the way we behave toward each other. No matter how upset or overwhelmed we get, we still make a very conscious effort to communicate and act in ways that are, at a bare minimum, respectful. And the value of autonomy means that while we can encourage and influence each other, in the end, we can't truly control each other and we don't want to force each other to do things that don't feel right to them, either. Each person in our family has autonomy over their body and their choices—even our kids (except in the cases where we need to do things that keep them healthy and safe). The final value, trust, helps us manage some of the feelings that can sometimes come up when we know we can't control other people. In our case, we trust each other to do the right thing for themselves *and* our family, and even if we make poor choices, we trust that we can address them, figure things out, and get through the tough consequences together.

When identifying your values, the most helpful way to approach it is with the constant awareness that you are a team. Take any issues that come up from a position of *we. How do* we *solve this problem?* Using terms like *us* and *we* includes both partners as key stakeholders. Even better, this "we mentality" subconsciously comforts both of you, reinforcing the team perspective and reminding you that you're in this together.

CONSIDERATIONS AND EXPECTATIONS

This month, you'll have enough just wrapping your head around what's happening. You may be embracing your new life, or you may be working on merely accepting the circumstances. It's all normal. Emotions will ebb and flow as you get used to your "new normal." Hopefully you've been taking advantage of the baby development YouTube series (see Resources, page 172) to see what developments your baby has made.

We were both excited and overwhelmed with the sheer thought of what needed to be done. But we always made room for fun and together time. We took walks during the day and snapped pictures with our new camera. But there were a few adjustments. For example, we loved to go on a midday sushi run before Rachel got pregnant. Since sushi is not recommended during pregnancy, that had to get cut out (although Rachel later found out that D'Anthony went on sushi runs without her!) along with several other foods that, if you google, you'll see are not appropriate for pregnancy. So this month, we began to accept things as they were, noticed areas in which changes were needed, and adjusted accordingly.

Hormones, Moods, and Feelings

At certain times during our pregnancies, we both found our feelings fluctuating up and down from day to day. This is normal—it's a lot to process. For the pregnant person, hormones may also play a role in feelings, and even mood swings, which are marked by a quick, drastic transition from one mood to another. When this happens, it can help for the non-birthing partner to rationalize this aberration as a result of pregnancy and not take it personally.

In His Words

Rachel and I were sitting in the living room watching television as we typically do on a weeknight. I casually grabbed the remote and turned the volume down. Then I proceeded to put the remote back where I got it. For some reason, that was the worst move that I could've ever made. Rachel was *not* a fan of that action. At the time of writing this book, I still have no idea what happened or why she got upset. But I set a rule for myself that I believe will help non-birthing partners: *Anything that seems absolutely out of character, classify as a mood swing due to pregnancy and don't take it personally.*

You may also find that your feelings leave you deep in thought, wondering how to act in response. Since our first child, Taj, was an unplanned pregnancy, we had a lot to talk about regarding who we should tell and how quickly we should tell them. We were apprehensive about telling people because we weren't married and didn't want to be judged by those who believed we should have been married before having a child. This weighed heavily on us.

If you're struggling with this sort of issue (or any other), know that you're not alone. We knew it would be difficult to share with some people in our world. We decided to first share the news with a couple of family members and close friends who we knew would be excited for us. They became our support system—they gave us a boost of confidence with every "Congratulations" or "I'm so happy for you." After so much support from people close to us, we felt ready enough to engage with those who might have opposed the timing of our pregnancy. You know who your support system is. Lean on that system as much as you can. Share the news and let their positive energy and excitement be a part of you, because that will raise you up.

Managing Pregnancy Side Effects

For us, month three meant the peak of nausea and sickness. Sometimes it lasted all day, while other times not at all. We had to figure out ways to manage the side effects. Rachel was often drained and had little to no energy, even if she slept all day. D'Anthony took full responsibility in suggesting when Rachel should rest. If you are the non-birthing partner, know that your partner may be torn between wanting to do things they normally do and feeling limited by their side effects. This is where you can step in with some emo deposits. If they lament that they don't have the energy to start their spring garden, surprise them with a few countertop herbs to care for. If you and your partner go on a daily walk, try to stop and rest along the way before the point where they usually get tired. A little empathy will likely reveal all kinds of ideas.

Workplace Considerations

Legally, companies with 15 or more employees cannot discriminate against employees who become pregnant, so, technically, you do not have to share your pregnancy news with your workplace. Although this is a federal law, review your company's HR manual to familiarize yourself with its specific policies regarding pregnant employees. However, depending on your job requirements and your pregnancy side effects and changes, it may be a good idea to share this information earlier rather than later. If you do decide to share the news before it becomes physically obvious, there are a few things to consider.

WHY AND WHEN SHOULD I SHARE THE NEWS? If your job has physical requirements, such as lifting or traveling, your pregnancy could result in physical limitations and prevent you from performing your normal job duties. Sickness or fatigue could impact your attendance or response time. The timing of your delivery and subsequent leave could conflict with major job-related activities. Consider these and any other reasons you may have for needing to share news of your pregnancy. Generally speaking, once you near the point at which you need any accommodations made, you'll want to inform your workplace. If you don't require any accommodations, then it's fine to tell your employer whenever you are comfortable doing so.

WHO SHOULD I SHARE THE NEWS WITH? If sharing the news is tied to a request for accommodations, then the people you share with are likely those who need to approve those accommodations. You may also choose to disclose in confidence to one or two trusted people who can maybe help you out at work. Who you share with is dependent on your relationships at work and how comfortable you are with sharing.

First Prenatal Screening

This month brings the first of various screenings and tests that will occur throughout your pregnancy. The first screening is an optional genetic test called nuchal translucency (NT), which occurs between weeks ten and thirteen and tests for the risk of Down syndrome and other chromosomal disorders. The screening includes a blood test and an ultrasound to visually measure the back of the baby's neck.

This is a clear moment to align on shared values. Together, discuss whether to conduct optional screenings and determine what testing you want performed. This particular test is not invasive, but there are other potential tests that could require an internal test, depending on the circumstances. Also, you'll want to discuss whether the tests results would matter to you in a way that would alter the way you treat or plan for the pregnancy.

Screenings and tests can become stressful if you consider all the what-if scenarios, so be sure to support each other through these stages. The best guidance is to remember that these technologies are available to provide information, and most babies are born healthy, so let this reassurance help you stay positive and think happy thoughts.

WEEKS 9–13

When Couples Face an Impasse

> Rachel and I disagreed on what to name our daughter, Aaliyah, for about eight and a half months. After suggesting a few names that got quickly shut down, I responded, "I feel insignificant when you quickly dismiss the names I come up with." Though we continued to disagree, the disagreement no longer put a strain on our relationship because I presented how I was feeling, and Rachel acknowledged my feelings.
>
> —— D'ANTHONY

Even the best relationships encounter challenges. Whether you've known your partner for ten years or six months before this pregnancy, there will be conflicts. Those conflicts may create other conflicts, and we're here to tell you that this is all normal. But what do you do when you simply cannot come to an agreement?

RESPECT EACH OTHER'S INDIVIDUALITY. First, keep in mind that your relationship doesn't have to be sacrificed over differences of opinions. You care about each other, and these differences don't define either of you—they're simply your respective independent thoughts and feelings. Surely you didn't choose each other because you were exactly alike!

USE "I" STATEMENTS. You can prevent disagreements from snowballing into new disagreements by approaching them with care. For example, when disagreeing over things like baby names or what genetic testing to do, try to use statements that begin with "I" to help your partner see your perspective. "I" statements work well because they focus on the issue without sparking defensiveness. An example of an "I" statement is "I feel this emotion when this happens."

CONTINUED

FIND COMMON GROUND. Would you rather be right or happy? Remember that the goal of an argument or disagreement is not to "win" but to find common ground and build off that until you find a resolution. During our name selection process, we agreed that we wanted a somewhat unique name. That became our common ground; from there, we could find solutions based on that criterion.

STAY ON POINT. Sometimes, arguments start about one thing and then digress into arguments over unrelated issues or old grudges. In our case, we would start debating baby names, but one comment would lead to another, and before you knew it, we'd be discussing some unresolved issue from months earlier. This is because we didn't focus on the exact reason why we were upset or concerned in the moment. It would have helped to zero in on the subject at hand—and stay there. We clearly had a few old issues to clean up and put to rest, which we did—in another conversation.

KNOW WHEN TO TAKE A BREAK. If you see an argument start to escalate, hit the brakes and commit to circling back later after you've had some time to cool off. For example, one of you could say, "Hey, I love you but things are getting heated. Let's take a break before one of us says something they'll regret." There's no rule that conflicts need to be solved in one sitting, and it's a lot easier to communicate with respect and compassion when both parties are feeling rested and emotionally resourced.

DIVIDE AND CONQUER

This month is still mostly about settling into the changes that your pregnancy has brought into your relationship. Don't overwhelm yourselves; instead, start prioritizing things as they come up. Non-birthing partners, see what parts of the workload you can shift onto your plate. Whether your partner is facing emotional and/or physical changes, your increased support is vital as you get through the final month of a sensitive first trimester.

This month includes more research and planning of activities. It'll also give you both an opportunity to practice using your shared values to guide decisions.

TIME-SENSITIVE

- Check if the pregnant person needs to disclose their pregnancy to their workplace

- Determine if your current home has enough space for the baby and where the baby will sleep

RESEARCH AND DISCUSS

- Parental-leave policies

- Nursery theme ideas

- Pregnancy announcement ideas

- Weekly baby development video (see Resources, page 172)

SCHEDULE AND PLAN

- Regular bedtime to get more sleep

- Relaxation activities

- Couple check-ins

ADDITIONAL

_____

_____

_____

_____

_____

_____

_____

DECIDE TOGETHER

Use these sheets to help you get on the same page when you're facing a tricky decision, like choosing a name or figuring out childcare.

YOUR PROBLEM OR DESIRED GOAL: _____

_____

What's important to Partner A?	What's important to Partner B?

Circle the top one to three things that matter most to you. Take turns explaining to your partner why your circled items are important to you. Then take some time separately to research and brainstorm solutions. List all your ideas, even wild or unusual ones.

_____

_____

_____

_____

_____

_____

List any factors that will impact your decision. This is where you set reasonable boundaries (time, cost, effort, etc.) about your possible solutions.

_____

_____

_____

_____

_____

_____

_____

_____

Partner A's short list	Partner B's short list

Discuss which solution is best for your relationship. Can you come to an enthusiastic agreement?

OUR FINAL DECISION: _____

PART TWO

THE SECOND TRIMESTER

Screenings and Meetings

Welcome to the second trimester! With all the responsibilities and serious consider-ations that come along with pregnancy, it can be lots of fun, too. Weeks 14 to 17 may provide a burst of energy and carefree planning that inspire you and your partner. Activities like selecting names, planning for photo ops and parties, maybe a possible getaway? Anything you do to bring levity will reset you, both individually and as a couple.

WHAT'S PHYSICALLY HAPPENING

Month four is a turning point for many reasons—the chances of miscarriage are greatly reduced after the first trimester, nausea should subside, and energy levels often begin to rebound.

This month, your baby now has eyelids, eyelashes, eyebrows, hair, and even nails! Their genitalia has formed, but unless you opt for an early blood test, you'll have to wait another month for the ultrasound to know the sex. In terms of size, a common comparison this month is an avocado.

The pregnant person is typically able to return to most normal activities. Every pregnancy is different, and so there may still be some lingering fatigue and nausea.

In Her Words

At this point with Taj, I was able to take a trip to Seattle to spend the weekend with friends and even went to a SoulCycle class. On the contrary, with Aaliyah, I would have never made it through a SoulCycle class, but I was able to make several trips to the store to shop for Christmas decorations. I spaced these trips out; short outings to one or two stores a day, as I was still tired and not back to full strength. After being sick, it felt so good to get out of the house and just get some fresh air.

Ideally, the non-birthing partner will continue to maintain the "heavy lifting" part of things and limit the stress on the pregnant person. This is especially true during holidays. Thanksgiving occurred in month four while pregnant with Aaliyah, and we hosted at our home with some family in attendance. Normally Rachel would have done all the cooking. Instead, D'Anthony found a caterer and had all the food delivered and set up, so when we woke up on Thanksgiving everything was already done. It was a great feeling for Rachel to not have that responsibility for a major holiday.

TEAM TOOLBOX

This Month's Strategy: Navigating Seas of Information

It seems like the pregnancy to-do list grows quickly from the first month to the second. Between doctor appointments, finances to manage, and childcare considerations, all these major tasks can get overwhelming. This month we'll focus on organization and systems. We put some systems in place that made things a bit easier for us to manage, and hopefully you can benefit, also.

APPOINTMENTS. It got very confusing for us to text each other reminders of scheduled appointments, so in addition to sharing our work calendars with each other, we also set up a joint Gmail account and shared that calendar, making sure alert notifications were turned on. We put all the appointments on that calendar and set a few reminders throughout the week.

INFORMATION MANAGEMENT. If you google the phrase *pregnancy symptoms*, I'm sure you will get a billion search results. As a newly pregnant couple, you may be overwhelmed and frustrated at the amount of conflicting information that you may read. We get it. A practical strategy for not getting overwhelmed is to set a timer for how long to spend researching a topic. This will ensure you don't get lost in a YouTube black hole. Pay attention to each other and encourage breaks if your partner is lingering too long or relying too much on the internet. Truth is, between all the information that you're going to get from your OB-GYN, plus what you are going to read in books or apps, and the unsolicited information that you will receive from friends and family, it's more than anyone needs.

In His Words

Rachel was craving a hamburger and fries, so I made a run to a local hamburger joint. While standing in line, I sparked a casual conversation with the guy behind me. I told him my wife was pregnant and he said, "Make sure she doesn't eat too many potatoes." I can't confirm why my burger-line-mate decided to give me this kind of advice, but the point is, there will be all types of information presented to you. People are often being very genuine and trying to be helpful when they present information. But *potatoes*?

In the end, it's best not to let unsolicited opinions be a driving force behind your decisions, or get stuck on everything you read. When you read something, consider the source. And then let the experts verify it. Here are some places you might turn for sound guidance:

HEALTHCARE PROVIDERS. When it comes to reliable information, the very first source to rely on is your healthcare provider. Any time we had a concern, we'd quickly skim through internet results before jotting the question down in our Notes app and present all our questions at the next doctor appointment.

MICRO- AND MIDLEVEL BLOGGERS. Smaller content creators in the family space are often good resources for information, as they tend to share unscripted and relatable experiences. Through their words, you're bound to uncover some nuggets of wisdom that can help you and your partner through your own unique pregnancy. Don't necessarily believe it all; just take what's good for you and leave the rest.

TRUSTED FRIENDS AND FAMILY. Folks in your family and friends circle will surely want to offer you their guidance. We got lucky: When we were pregnant with Taj, three of our close friends were also pregnant, all due within months of one another. It was relieving to share similar experiences and bounce ideas off one another, but we learned it's important not to expect the exact same experiences or get freaked out if something different happened to you. And some advice you receive may be outdated, misguided, or completely ridiculous; if so, you can free yourself of this conversation with a simple nod in a "duly noted" way and proceed as you wish.

CONSIDERATIONS AND EXPECTATIONS

This month, you may be more comfortable with openly sharing the news of your pregnancy beyond close friends or family. You may choose to do an announcement on social media or call some friends you haven't spoken to in a while and let them know that you're pregnant.

We love traveling, and month four was a good time for us to plan a couple of getaways. We took a trip to Seattle for a Seahawks football game. Amazingly, twenty thousand screaming fans packed into "the Home of the 12s" didn't cause Rachel any issues or discomfort. This trip was an awesome experience and a great opportunity for us to reconnect after so much that was happening in the months prior: the shock of being pregnant, and navigating all the information and responsibilities that come along with being pregnant, not to mention finding a way to tell the people closest to us *and* moving in together. It was the first time in several months that we felt like a normal couple who just *happened* to be pregnant.

Screenings and Tests

Another genetic testing option will likely be offered to you, generally known as the multiple markers test. Done between weeks 15 and 20, this is a continuation of the testing from the previous month. It is a blood draw that will test for similar disorders as the previous month, but with both tests being done, the doctors can more accurately determine any potential risks. It does not provide definitive results as to whether the disorder exists; just the likelihood of it occurring. For pregnant people 35 years and older, like we were while pregnant with Aaliyah, genetic testing will be highly encouraged. We did the first trimester screening with both pregnancies, but did the second trimester genetic screening only with Aaliyah.

The Birth Team

You may be settled into the idea of receiving your care and delivery by your OB-GYN. This is the most common approach to pregnancy and delivery care, and as such, you'll be under the care of a medical professional with specialized training in this area. However, there are other options for both prenatal care and delivery, such as midwives and doulas. Depending on your healthcare plan, you may be able to have their services covered, too.

Midwives are trained health professionals who provide pregnant women with obstetric and gynecological care, including primary care, prenatal care, childbirth, postpartum care, and even care of the newborn. A midwife is often chosen by people who wish to deliver their baby at home, as well as those who seek an unmedicated childbirth (without an epidural).

Doulas provide the pregnant mother with education and physical and emotional support throughout pregnancy and delivery. While not a medical professional, a doula attends childbirth education and birth-doula training and observes deliveries before receiving certification. Research has shown that expectant mothers placed with a doula had better birth outcomes than those who chose not to work with a prebirth assistant.

Who you choose to turn to for care is a personal decision. If you do your homework and find someone you trust, any one or all of these professionals can prove invaluable in your journey.

Names, Parties, Photos, and Fun

> If you're anything like my wife, she didn't want to spend money on maternity clothes, but I reassured her that she deserved to do so. Helping Rachel shop and enthusiastically telling her that each outfit looked great didn't take much effort on my part, but small emo deposits like that go a long way in making your partner feel good about themself and you.
>
> —D'ANTHONY

With all the seriousness and responsibilities around pregnancy, it's easy to lose sight of the fact that you and your partner are creating a person! A person you will bond with, talk to, and build a home for. What better cause for celebration? Let's talk about some of the details.

CLOTHING. If you're the pregnant partner, your body may be changing, and people may be starting to notice that you are expecting. It may be time to go and look at some new clothes. Buying clothes for what seems like a limited amount of time may seem frustrating, but keep in mind that you'll likely wear them for some time after the baby's born, as well. Depending on your budget, options can range from consignment-shop finds to high-end maternity-boutique clothing. You can reach out to your friend network or online sources like your local Facebook Buy Nothing group to see who's unloading their clothes for free or cheap. There are even clothing hacks to extend the time you wear your current clothes before having to buy new ones. For example, a small ponytail holder can help hold your jeans together when you can no longer button them—Amazon even sells jean extenders for this exact purpose!

CONTINUED

NAMES. Unsurprisingly, you're going to need to give your baby a name once they arrive. Surprisingly, we forgot about names while we were in the thick of it all. Use this time to start "negotiations" if you don't have a name already picked out. Before Aaliyah was Aaliyah, we picked out about 25 different names that we were sure we'd agree on—we were wrong. We did a deep dive into the meaning of names to find something that represented us both, while still allowing our children to have their own unique and meaningful identity.

PHOTOS. Take all the photos you can! This can get away from you; we understand. During our first pregnancy, with Taj, photos seemed like a luxury; something that required spare time and energy (two things that don't often go together during pregnancy). Looking back, we agreed that we didn't take as many photos as we should have. Please, set aside time to take photos at home—you won't regret it. Casual ones are as good as staged ones; a random snapshot of real life in action, after dinner or during a lazy day on the couch, can make for the most treasured memories down the line.

IF YOU CAN, MOVE BEYOND SELFIES. A professional photographer is a wonderful way to capture your pregnancy. Enlist someone you know, or just look on social media. For example, we went on Instagram and searched #AtlantaMaternityPhotographer. You could do the same (replacing Atlanta with the city you live in). You'll see a lot of options and creative ideas, and from this, you can start to decide what you want your style to be. This was a fun exercise for us at this point in our pregnancy, as it gave us months to think about what we liked and didn't like and decide what kind of mood we wanted to capture for our pregnancy photos.

BABY BONDING. It's not too early to bond with your baby! By week 20, you can often hear baby's heartbeat with a stethoscope, but if you can't wait, grab an at-home fetal doppler. A doppler is used to monitor the baby's heartbeat in the womb. There are home versions of these that are quite inexpensive and a fun investment. They provide another opportunity for you and your partner to connect with each other and your baby during the pregnancy. Grabbing the doppler anytime we wanted to hear our baby kept us grounded during the whole pregnancy experience.

PARTY PLANNING. This is around the time you're given the option to find out the sex of your baby. As you've probably seen, there are only about a million ways to reveal this information. Picture six-layer cakes, streamers, and rapturous audiences of hundreds of people. Or picture the opposite, with an envelope and just the two of you at the kitchen table, or holding hands while watching the sonographer do an ultrasound at the doctor's office. If you're not into gender-reveal parties, some popular alternatives include pregnancy reveal, name reveal, "chosen family" reveal, and even birthstone or zodiac sign reveal. It's all up to you and how you want to celebrate your exciting news with your favorite people.

DIVIDE AND CONQUER

The to-do list for this month is a mix of practical and fun—the theme for most of the second trimester. The items on this list will inevitably lead to a lot of internet searches, so be sure to use the strategies shared in this month's Team Toolbox (page 61). Set aside additional time for the couple check-in this month, perhaps to reflect on the first trimester. You can also use the check-ins to discuss the results of things you're researching and get a sense of how each partner feels about the information that's discovered and shared.

TIME-SENSITIVE

- Genetic testing (if doing)
- Maternity or pregnancy clothes

RESEARCH AND DISCUSS

- Names
- Gender reveal
- Parental leave
- Childcare options
- Weekly baby development video (see Resources, page 172)

SCHEDULE AND PLAN

- Exercise
- Time to have fun together
- Couple check-in

ADDITIONAL

_____
_____
_____
_____
_____
_____
_____
_____
_____
_____
_____
_____
_____
_____
_____
_____
_____
_____
_____
_____
_____
_____
_____
_____
_____

DECIDE TOGETHER

Use these sheets to help you get on the same page when you're facing a tricky decision, like choosing a name or figuring out childcare.

YOUR PROBLEM OR DESIRED GOAL: _____

_____

What's important to Partner A?	What's important to Partner B?

Circle the top one to three things that matter most to you. Take turns explaining to your partner why your circled items are important to you. Then take some time separately to research and brainstorm solutions. List all your ideas, even wild or unusual ones.

_____

_____

_____

_____

_____

_____

_____

List any factors that will impact your decision. This is where you set reasonable boundaries (time, cost, effort, etc.) about your possible solutions.

_____

_____

_____

_____

_____

_____

_____

_____

Partner A's short list	Partner B's short list

Discuss which solution is best for your relationship. Can you come to an enthusiastic agreement?

OUR FINAL DECISION: _____

Checklists and Classes

For the past few months, you and your partner have been adjusting together and individually to the world of pregnancy, processing more thoughts and emotions than perhaps ever before. The taxing anxiety around taking tests, planning your budgetary and household strategies, and processing all the changes happening all play a part. This month we talk about routine testing, dive deeper into parental-leave considerations, and discuss how to carve out a little room for yourself.

WHAT'S PHYSICALLY HAPPENING

Whoa, what was *that?* This month may bring the first feelings of baby movements. These movements can only be felt internally by the pregnant person, not yet by the non-birth partner. But this is where it starts. These subtle feelings are most commonly described as fluttering, butterflies, or gas bubbles, and you may also hear them referred to as quickening. Not every pregnant person will feel or recognize these movements.

Your baby now has hair, and all body parts can clearly be seen by an ultrasound, which will be done during the anatomy scan. We recommend you both be present to share in this exciting moment, regardless of whether you decide to find out the sex or not. The view is tremendous.

By the end of the month, the baby will be the size of a grapefruit. If you haven't started showing already, you will likely not make it out of this month without people starting to notice the growth.

In Her Words

This was the month I shared Taj's pregnancy with coworkers, because my clothes no longer hid my growing belly. My energy was up, and I felt more familiar with how my body was responding to things now. During this month, while pregnant with Taj, I planned and threw a birthday party for D'Anthony, and while pregnant with Aaliyah, I spent time decorating our house for Christmas. It felt good to be back in the game.

TEAM TOOLBOX

This Month's Strategy: Intentional Self-Care

At this point, you and your partner may have been spending a lot of time together, brainstorming, rationalizing, planning, anticipating, and even worrying. As the pregnant partner's body begins to take on the weight of the growing baby and uterus, the non-birthing partner has likely taken on a good amount of responsibility trying to lighten their partner's load. As the non-birthing partner, it may seem like there is a never-ending cycle of tasks to complete while possibly suppressing your own emotions in an attempt to relieve your partner of any unnecessary stress. You've been immersed in a cycle of mental exercises and emotional containment that you may not even realize because of all the excitement surrounding the pregnancy. It's okay to communicate your needs, and it's important for both of you to engage in self-care.

This month's strategy for both partners is, in fact, to focus on self-care. Some alone time away from your partner can be restorative, too. For the non-birthing person, this can be the perfect time to practice self-care strategies, as your partner is most likely feeling better, freeing you up a bit to take time to yourself.

As the pregnant person, this time to yourself can be invaluable as well. It gives you time to reflect on everything that has happened as well as what's waiting for you ahead, and since your early-pregnancy side effects have hopefully subsided, ideally you can reflect with a clear mind.

Self-care isn't an automatic response for everyone. As a couple, we learned that self-care and alone time becomes more approachable when it's brought up by the other person. For example, the non-birthing person might suggest that their partner get a pedicure or a pregnancy massage, or even just a bubble bath or a nap. That can be a powerful suggestion that gives the pregnant person's subconscious "permission" to clear their mind of distractions for the time being. By being encouraged to take time to relax and care for themself, the pregnant partner is relieved of the burden of feeling that they should be doing something "more productive" or preparing for the baby's arrival. And vice versa: As the pregnant person, you can reassure your partner that you're doing fine today, so why not have them take some time for themselves.

In His Words

During this time, Rachel would occasionally mention she was going to leave the house to clear her head. At first, that triggered something in me, thinking that she might be overwhelmed. This concern would lead me to check in, making sure she was okay and asking if there's anything else I could take off her plate. She reassured me that she just wanted some alone time, and this helped me realize that I could take some time for myself, because I knew she would understand and would not mind if I did the same.

Giving each other permission to take a break and treat yourselves is important because you have both been carrying more responsibility than before in your relationship. Support each other by encouraging your partner to go do something they enjoy for a while. Without your unprovoked blessing, it may never happen.

When both partners focus on self-care and get some alone time, it enables everyone to refresh and make more space for each other. This was a winning strategy for us, and a perfect one to implement during this month.

CONSIDERATIONS AND EXPECTATIONS

This month involves a few routine screenings to see how things are coming along. We'll share our experience on anatomy screening and genetic testing and a big-picture overview of what it all means. It's also a good time to begin mapping out your parental-leave benefits so you understand the time and compensation available to you after your baby is born.

Anatomy Screening

When it comes to testing and screenings, there are a good number of tests that we would have never thought of had the options not been introduced to us. Pregnancy is exciting, but it seemed for us that when we went through the several tests, a level of paranoia was also introduced. This paranoia is completely normal and expected; however, there is no need to panic—these screenings are standard tests that they offer to everyone. For some tests, if results come back unfavorable, the issue can be fixed before birth or the necessary resources can be put in place to address the issue after birth. We found comfort in knowing that these tests provided an opportunity to get in front of any underlining issues.

The anatomy scan typically allows us to identify the sex of the baby; it also enables doctors to review the anatomy of the baby, because at this point the baby is developed enough to identify normalcies or irregularities with body parts. If any abnormalities are detected, this early detection can allow for advance planning.

Genetic Testing

As mentioned on page 63, genetic testing is meant to identify irregularities or confirm normalcies from a genetic point of view. We take all these tests in hopes that nothing is wrong. At first, we thought that if something *was* wrong, it would've been devastating to us. Though we lived in that state for quite a while, as we got more mature in our thinking, we found comfort in knowing that we would be able to get ahead of anything that *did* go wrong.

In His Words

While pregnant with Aaliyah, Rachel did some additional genetic testing. We hadn't done this with Taj and assumed there'd be no issues, but the test came back positive for one genetic disorder. The team recommended testing me, too, which caught me off guard. It turned out I also carry the gene. We met virtually with the genetic counselor. As Rachel and I sat there on the Zoom call, all we could think about was how to get in front of this. In a calming voice, the genetic counselor told us that the configuration of this gene is crucial, and that it just so happened that the configuration of my gene did *not* result in a high probability of the disorder occurring in Aaliyah. Whew.

So our hard-earned advice to you: If you choose to take this genetic test, resist the urge to jump to any conclusions until you have your results. The medical world is complex, and for anything out of the ordinary to happen, the science needs to line up in a very particular way. Try not to cause more stress than needed by spiraling out over the what-ifs. Stay positive. Keep busy with fun activities. Remain distant from the internet-research rabbit hole. And, of course, do frequent check-ins to stay in tune with each other.

Parental Leave

It may seem early, but now's the perfect time to begin researching your parental leave and discussing your post-birth plan. Questions to investigate might include:

- How much time off do each of you get from work?

- Do you have to take the time off all at once?

- Is it fully paid, partially paid, or unpaid time?

- If the time is partially paid or unpaid, how long you can afford the pay reduction?

- Once you return to work, who will be responsible for the baby during working hours?

- Do either of you want to stay home with the baby? Is this feasible?

- Are there friends or family who might be interested in helping care for the baby?

- If day care, which day care will they attend?

- What are the day care costs versus income; is it worth it?

In Her Words

D'Anthony and I were blessed to have my mom and then his grand-mother, both retired, come stay with us to help with Taj when he was first born. D'Anthony's grandmother came and lived with us for three months and took care of Taj while we were at work. After she left, we transferred him into a day care program, but while it lasted, it was reassuring to know he was in such loving hands—and the experi-ences provided a priceless bonding experience.

When Finances Feel Tight

> I constantly ordered DoorDash while pregnant with Aaliyah because I was nauseated and desperate to find something I could keep down, but this came at a price. In fact, we realized it had led to an additional $800 in food expenses on top of our regular monthly budget! Definitely track your expenses so you avoid eye-popping surprises like this one.
>
> —RACHEL

Let's address the elephant in the room: Having a baby is expensive!

No matter what your budget, planning to the best of your ability is the best way to reduce the stress of increased expenses. There are two ranges worth planning for: during pregnancy and after pregnancy. We discussed a little of both in chapter 2 (page 33) regarding taking stock of your current finances so you can effectively plan for the future.

One of the first activities we did after finding out that we were pregnant with Taj was sit down and list all our household expenses line by line in a spreadsheet. This was eye-opening—you don't realize how much you spend on certain things until you list it all out! This allowed us to see where we could reduce expenses to put toward baby-related expenses.

We also did a little research to determine average costs for things like diapers, wipes, baby food, childcare, prenatal care, and delivery (both vaginal and C-section). While not a complete picture, it provides good enough estimates to help you begin to budget.

Here are a few simple cost-cutting actions.

COOK INSTEAD OF ORDERING TAKEOUT OR GOING OUT TO DINNER. Though it may be difficult for the pregnant person to adhere to this suggestion (especially when they do the cooking), cooking and eating leftovers goes a long way in helping you save.

One simple strategy is to "cook once, eat twice" by doubling the amount you cook at a time and freezing the leftovers.

SEEK OUT HAND-ME-DOWN BABY GEAR AND CLOTHES. Some of our favorite baby items for Taj were hand-me-downs from friends. We had a Pack 'n Play that a friend had used with two of her children, and it was the only place Taj would sleep—for hours! He hated the pricey baby swing, but it seemed that he loved all the free, used items. Your local Facebook Buy Nothing group will likely have tons of free baby clothes and gear—often in great condition.

CHECK IF THE HOSPITAL OFFERS FREE BIRTHING (OR OTHER PREGNANCY-RELATED) CLASSES. Most hospitals offer free classes for those planning to deliver in the hospital. The classes may be in-person or virtual.

SET UP A MANAGEABLE PAYMENT PLAN WITH HEALTHCARE PROVIDERS. Most hospitals will offer the option of a payment plan leading up to the birth and again after delivery. They also have financial offices that can offer support if you cannot afford the delivery costs. We were on a monthly payment plan for both Taj and Aaliyah.

CONSIDER BREASTFEEDING OR CHESTFEEDING. This is a very personal decision. We can tell you this: For us, there were many benefits to breastfeeding; not the least of which is the ability to produce milk at the perfect temperature at any time (including 3:00 a.m.!). If you are interested in nursing and are able to do so without difficulty, it can eliminate the need to purchase baby formula and wash a ton of bottles. However, the time and energy required to nurse means there will be less time for other activities, be it household chores or tasks for your day job. In our case, Aaliyah refused to take a bottle for seven months, which meant all feeding responsibilities fell on Rachel. Depending on your situation, the decision to

CONTINUED

nurse may be a complicated one. See Resources (page 173) for more on this.

MAKE HOMEMADE BABY FOOD AND FREEZE IT. Once your baby moves into the world of purees, another option is to make your baby's food rather than buying it premade. One sweet potato can make several servings for a fraction of the cost of a jar of sweet potato puree. This does add another responsibility, and you'll probably need a high-speed blender, so weigh the options.

LOOK INTO POSSIBLE CHILDCARE SUPPORT BY FAMILY/ FRIENDS. Consider whether you have any family or friends who are willing and able to care for your baby when/if you must return to work, and remember that any amount of time helps.

DIVIDE AND CONQUER

This month is a planning month. It's time to prepare for the second half of the pregnancy, when things will get busier. As always, these are just our recommendations to help minimize the stress from a long list of to-dos between now and the end of the pregnancy.

TIME-SENSITIVE

- Decide whether to find out the baby's sex
- Share news of pregnancy as needed/desired

RESEARCH AND DISCUSS

- Parental leave and childcare
- Financial plan for baby needs (short and long term)
- Weekly baby development video (see Resources, page 172)

SCHEDULE AND PLAN

- Self-care time for *both* partners
- Birthing classes
- Couple check-in

ADDITIONAL

_____

_____

_____

_____

_____

_____

_____

_____

_____

_____

_____

_____

_____

_____

_____

_____

DECIDE TOGETHER

Use these sheets to help you get on the same page when you're facing a tricky decision, like choosing a name or figuring out childcare.

YOUR PROBLEM OR DESIRED GOAL: _____

_____

What's important to Partner A?	What's important to Partner B?

Circle the top one to three things that matter most to you. Take turns explaining to your partner why your circled items are important to you. Then take some time separately to research and brainstorm solutions. List all your ideas, even wild or unusual ones.

_____

_____

_____

_____

_____

_____

List any factors that will impact your decision. This is where you set reasonable boundaries (time, cost, effort, etc.) about your possible solutions.

_____

_____

_____

_____

_____

_____

_____

_____

Partner A's short list	Partner B's short list

Discuss which solution is best for your relationship. Can you come to an enthusiastic agreement?

OUR FINAL DECISION: _____

Registry, Babymoon, and Pediatricians

Month six is a tactical month. We won't just be talking about how to reframe your thoughts or enjoy your time. This month you have a to-do list to conquer! We have some helpful strategies that we used to construct a baby registry that worked for us and creative thoughts on planning a baby-moon. You'll want to get started researching pediatricians for your baby. And if it's on your mind, we'll discuss intimacy and how you can "meet in the middle" during these busy and emotional times.

WHAT'S PHYSICALLY HAPPENING

This month will likely involve more physical activity from both the pregnant partner and the baby. At this point, the best way to keep your body feeling good is to be active every day. We would try to take a walk each day—nothing intense—literally just strolled and talked for a couple of blocks. Based on how you feel and how active you were prior to the pregnancy, you can increase your activity level; just get your doctor's consent.

Toward the end of this month, your baby will begin to open their eyes and make larger movements. If the mild fluttering didn't catch your attention the previous month, this month you may begin to feel your baby move. There's some good growth happening here; by the end of the month, your baby will be the size of an eggplant.

In Her Words

Your baby bump may start getting in the way. With Taj, this was the month that sleeping became uncomfortable for me. Finding the best sleeping position and location may take a bit of trial and error. I didn't sleep very well at night in the bed; I slept better taking naps on the couch during the day—not ideal, but I knew what worked for me. Pregnancy pillows are popular, but they weren't comfortable for me. Using multiple regular pillows and positioning them in front and in back of me worked better. Hang in there—you'll find your ideal position.

TEAM TOOLBOX

This Month's Strategy: Outsources and Resources

People are capable of accomplishing many tasks at once. I mean, we simultaneously walk, talk, and think. We process signals in our minds that we don't even consciously pay attention to. Likewise, living in a household together involves multiple responsibilities: cooking, cleaning, planning, bookkeeping, home repairs, having fun, giving each other the support and love they need, etc. Many things require our direct attention. For us, it became too much, so we tried to figure out which tasks we might be able to outsource. And we'd like for you to ask yourselves the same question. Take a look at your finances versus the time that you spend on various "to-do" list tasks around the home. What are the things that you wouldn't mind paying for if it meant you'd reduce stress and gain back some time and energy?

In Her Words

We took a long, hard look at this question, and we determined that our weak point is keeping the house clean. We decided, for the sake of our productivity and well-being, to hire a cleaning company to help us out. D'Anthony battled with the thought of someone coming into our home to clean for us, because it was completely opposite from how we were raised. It took some convincing on my part. We realized it would help us work better together, give us more free time, and relieve stress, and we looked at our budget to see where we could make sacrifices to make this work. For us, this decision has been worth it; the relief we feel after the house gets cleaned has been amazing.

Figure out what areas will relieve the most stress in your home. Maybe it's food shopping. If your supermarket offers pickup or delivery, consider taking advantage of this service. Any service fee is offset by the fact that you will avoid purchasing impulse items that you see in the store. You'll save more by shopping the sales in the online circular and comparing cost by weight between brands.

Don't be afraid to outsource the things that make your life easier. This kind of couple discovery may take some uncomfortable work for the both of you, like establishing what you're willing to sacrifice, wrapping your heads around the cost benefit, and releasing old beliefs about perceived extravagances. However, if you're willing to get through these uncomfortable discussions now, it can result in a big win for Team You in the long run.

In His Words

Rachel typically does all the cooking in our home, but cooking every night while pregnant is not fun, and Rachel could only stomach my scrambled eggs and pancakes for dinner so many times. We began to incorporate "takeout days" in addition to food delivery services for our groceries. Financially planning around this took some work, but since we determined together that it was best for us, it was just a matter of creating a plan, sticking to it, and basking in the success of it all.

CONSIDERATIONS AND EXPECTATIONS

Use this month as an opportunity to leverage your community for guidance and recommendations. If it takes a village to raise a child, then this is a great month to start thinking about the kind of village you'll need. This month also involves a test for gestational diabetes as well as some thoughts around building a useful baby registry, planning a babymoon, and choosing a pediatrician for the baby.

Gestational Diabetes Test

This month the pregnant person will be asked to take a one-hour glucose test to check for gestational diabetes, which is diabetes that shows up in a person who didn't have diabetes prior to pregnancy. You'll drink a sugary solution and then get blood drawn to measure your blood glucose. If your sugar levels are too high, you'll have to do a three-hour glucose test. In this case, you'll have to drink the sugary stuff once every hour and have your blood drawn every hour for three hours. Of course you'll want to avoid this hassle if you can, so we recommend doing a little research (see Resources, page 172, for more on this.).

If you test positive for gestational diabetes, you'll need to monitor your blood sugar levels, and your doctor will likely recommend a healthy diet and regular exercise.

In Her Words

While pregnant with Taj, I failed my one-hour glucose test because I ate several chocolate bars the night before my test and had to do the three-hour glucose test (which came back negative). So my advice: Try to avoid excessive sugars and carbs the night before and day of the test!

The Baby Registry

It's a great time to create a baby registry. You'll want to choose the store that fits your needs. Naturally, some stores have more variety than others, and variety is important because if your favorite baby store only has a small variety of baby items, your registry will get filled up very quickly if your gift-giving friends and family outweigh the number of baby items available. As a result, you may receive duplicate items or items you don't need.

Think about price range, bearing in mind the circle of friends who will be purchasing items from your baby registry. For friends with varying budgets, choosing a high-end boutique to house your registry may not be the best idea. We made registries at Target and Amazon because each site carried specific items we liked. Amazon was preferred by our guests, and we liked its ease of use, which allowed us to spend time together and simply check off items virtually that we needed.

The ideal baby list is intuitive: It has everything you need, as well as some things you may not think you need—until you need them. Talking with other parents about the baby items that work for them is a helpful way to build that intuition.

It also helps to think about the person who will be purchasing items for you. What do you think the first thing people like to purchase for new babies? Clothing, of course! No matter what the occasion, people like to gift clothing for babies, and some people buy these in addition to items they choose from your baby registry. With this in mind, we decided to not put any baby clothing on the registry, since we knew people would purchase clothes anyway. This gave us room to put more items on the registry that we absolutely needed.

There were a few items purchased from our registry that, in retrospect, we probably didn't need:

- Bottle warmer: We thought it was easier to put the bottle of milk in warm water and set a timer.

- Baby wipe warmer: A good idea in theory and very polite step to take for your baby, but they'll be okay with regular wipes.

- Baby mittens: We have never used these, even though we have a ton. Filing their nails works well to eliminate sharp edges.

- Baby shoes: They're cute. But your baby can't walk. And it takes a lot of work to put them on. Okay for a photo shoot or special occasion, but for day-to-day life, we vote for saving your energy.

- Bottle sterilizer: It's pretty much a bag that you put bottles in, and then you put the bag of bottles in the microwave. A pot of water does the same thing.

Babymoon

No matter your budget—yes, you can! (More on that soon.)

We had no idea what a babymoon was, but once we found out, we were definitely on board. A babymoon is a designated "vacation" that couples go on as their last hurrah together before the baby is born. It's a precious time to spend time together, connect with each other, and just relax right before things get even more hectic and busy with the arrival of a new baby!

You'll want to wait until after the pregnant person's nausea is pretty much nonexistent, but don't wait too long, because later in the pregnancy the baby will be large and taking up more space, which can become quite uncomfortable. So, if you plan a babymoon, it's ideal to plan to take it before you get to this point, and definitely well before your delivery date. It would *not* be ideal to go into labor eight hours away from the doctor you've been seeing for the past eight months.

There are countless locations you can go for a babymoon, by land or air. The preference is completely up to you; however, we were comfortable with a two- to three-hour drive from our hospital. This gave us peace of mind that we were away but not too far away in case something happened and we needed to cut the trip short. Depending on how far along you are, your doctor may restrict all flights.

Wherever you choose to go—boutique hotel, bed-and-breakfast, cabin in the woods, mountain vista, or lake house—pick a place you'll both enjoy and spend the time together. How long you stay is up to you; even a one-night stay can be surprisingly rejuvenating. The quality of your time is most important; in fact, we recommend leaving your phones in your pockets so you can really savor each other's company.

So now let's talk about budget. Nothing should stand in the way of you getting away as a couple. If finances are tight, consider a home swap with another family. Perhaps you have trusted friends who are also pregnant—see if they're interested in swapping homes for the weekend. Make it special for each other by leaving each other snacks and setting out the "good towels." If you're disciplined enough, you could also simply unplug and agree to have an intimate getaway in your own home, free of distractions and chores. Promise to leave the laundry, bills, and computer work alone for 24 hours, until your return to "reality."

The purpose of the babymoon is not to experience as much as you can before the baby comes; rather, it's just to spend quality time together. While we were on our babymoon, we made it a point to relax. We didn't have a lot planned: no organized activities and not much moving around, either. Just some strawberries, sparkling cider, and our favorite Netflix shows.

Choosing a Pediatrician

Much like choosing an OB-GYN or other healthcare provider, choosing your baby's primary health provider requires a combination of homework and good rapport. Check with your insurance carrier to see which local pediatricians are in-network. Then seek referrals—friends, family, trusted neighbors, and online community group members are priceless resources for word-of-mouth recommendations. Once you've found one or more pediatricians you'd like to meet, call and schedule a consultation. There's no commitment needed. You are simply trying to discern whether this provider is a good fit for you. Bring your questions and ask them. Things to ask might include:

- What's your position on [whatever issues are important to you]?

- What are your hours? Do you have weekend hours?

- Who covers for you when you're away?

- How many doctors or practitioners are in the practice? Can we request certain doctors?

- Do you support a parent's choice in vaccinating? Circumcising?

- Are you a parent?

- What is your perspective on childcare?

- How long have you been in practice?

- What hospitals do you have admitting rights at?

You might also ask open-ended questions, such as what they love about their job. These questions may reveal insights into the doctor's attitudes and personality that prove deciding factors in whether to go with them. Likewise, share your values and see how they respond. Are they patient? Responsive? Dismissive? Finally, if you decide at any point, for any reason, that this professional relationship is not working, know that you are absolutely free to move on to another provider who can better meet your needs.

Keeping Intimacy Alive

> **Sometimes I'd look at Rachel and think, Wow, she looks awesome. Her hair is curly. Her stomach is perfectly round. She's clearly mid-thought because she has her mid-thought face on. All of that is attractive to me. Meanwhile, she's thinking: I can't do anything with my hair. My stomach is so big; I'm uncomfortable. I have so much to do to prepare for this baby. Clearly, my thought process involved intimacy; hers did not.**
>
> **——D'ANTHONY**

Keeping intimacy alive during pregnancy takes communication, flexibility, and some trial and error—especially if you think one way and your partner thinks another. We both realized that, for a while, our sex life would be spent trying to get on the same page with each other.

For the non-birthing partner, it's important to expand the definition of intimacy. Since your pregnant partner is going through intense physical changes, it's kind of on you to adjust your definition of intimacy and realize it could range from intercourse to a simple caress. Both partners want something that connects them with the other. They want vulnerability. Being emotionally intimate—that is, completely vulnerable with your thoughts and your feelings—is just as intimate as being naked in the bedroom. It's just a different way of connecting.

For example, D'Anthony admits that there were times during pregnancy when he felt rejected, only to learn later it wasn't rejection; it was Rachel craving a different form of intimacy. If your pregnant partner comes up and lays their head on your chest, it's not necessarily an invitation or precursor to intercourse. If you are a non-birthing partner, we recommend letting your pregnant partner lead the way. This may be tough at first, especially if you tend to be the partner to initiate more often. But patience and emotional vulnerability, along with open communication, can deepen intimacy—including your sex life.

DIVIDE AND CONQUER

The remaining months are full of major tasks, so it will be more important than ever to remember to divide and conquer. The pregnant person will hopefully feel good and be up to helping a little more, so decide which tasks you each can do separately and which you can do together. Consider leaning on others, family or friends, to help both of you. Divide and conquer does not always have to be just between the couple, so invite your support system to join in to help for these remaining months. And, as always, these are suggestions, not requirements.

TIME-SENSITIVE

- Gestational diabetes test
- Birthing classes
- Baby registry

RESEARCH AND DISCUSS

- Babymoon
- Parental-leave plan and childcare
- Pediatrician
- Sleeping strategies with belly
- Weekly baby development video (see Resources, page 172)

SCHEDULE AND PLAN

- Baby shower
- Couple check-in

ADDITIONAL

_____

_____

_____

_____

_____

_____

_____

_____

_____

_____

_____

_____

_____

_____

_____

WEEKS 23–27

DECIDE TOGETHER

Use these sheets to help you get on the same page when you're facing a tricky decision, like choosing a name or figuring out childcare.

YOUR PROBLEM OR DESIRED GOAL: _____

_____

What's important to Partner A?	What's important to Partner B?

Circle the top one to three things that matter most to you. Take turns explaining to your partner why your circled items are important to you. Then take some time separately to research and brainstorm solutions. List all your ideas, even wild or unusual ones.

_____

_____

_____

_____

_____

_____

_____

List any factors that will impact your decision. This is where you set reasonable boundaries (time, cost, effort, etc.) about your possible solutions.

_____

_____

_____

_____

_____

_____

_____

_____

_____

Partner A's short list	Partner B's short list

Discuss which solution is best for your relationship. Can you come to an enthusiastic agreement?

OUR FINAL DECISION: _____

PART THREE

THE
THIRD
TRIMESTER

Birth Plans and Preferences

You're two-thirds of the way there! It's time for some birth planning; that is, determining your ideal birthing scenario. In this chapter, we'll provide ideas for how to work together to become more prepared for and capable of what's to come in the weeks and months ahead. You'll get to have a bit of fun, too, with things like setting up a nursery, filling your baby's closet with clothes, and surrounding yourself with love at a baby shower that engages your community and helps you celebrate your baby's nearing arrival.

WHAT'S PHYSICALLY HAPPENING

The third trimester brings yet another transition in feelings as your due date nears. This month will likely physically feel similar to month six, in that energy levels are probably pretty good. In fact, as delivery becomes more real, you may be more motivated to get stuff done or just get out and live life before your new addition arrives. If you're the pregnant partner, your baby will probably be more active and your belly will be bigger in month seven, so you will need to adjust for comfort more often. Just remember that every pregnancy is different, so don't be surprised if your baby moves less or more, or has days where you don't feel them as much. Some babies are definitely more active in utero than others.

This month, your baby will start storing fat to prepare for delivery and will be about the size of a butternut squash by the end of the month. Your baby's hearing is fully developed, so you may start to notice them reacting to sounds. When you notice a reaction, share this very special and intimate moment with your partner, so they can talk or read to the baby, play music, or sing songs.

In Her Words

I was pretty active during this month while pregnant with Taj. At work, I was in the peak of my busy season, so I was doing a lot of traveling and spent many long days on my feet. There were times that Taj seemed to be doing backflips in my belly as I was trying to settle into bed or sleep. As soon as D'Anthony would lean over and speak calmly to him, Taj would settle down. It was so cute and frustrating at the same time—I wish he'd have settled down for me!

TEAM TOOLBOX

This Month's Strategy: Finding Your Balance

Understanding your strengths in a relationship is pretty straightforward—you each know what you're good at. Those strengths may be the reason why you're in the relationship in the first place. Something about your strengths may have even caused you to overlook some of one another's weaknesses. But there comes a point in every relationship when those weaknesses emerge. Not because you're doing anything wrong, but because everyone has vulnerabilities.

Understanding and addressing your weaknesses/needs/vulnerabilities—whatever you want to call them—will help you transition to parenting more smoothly. One big concern we had before Taj was born was how we would get through the night once he arrived. We'd heard horror stories about sleepless parents, forced to stay up all night because the baby wouldn't let them sleep. In our case, we knew that Rachel needed her sleep at night. But Rachel also needed to breastfeed the baby. *If the baby wakes up at all hours of the night*, we thought, *what are we going to do?*

D'Anthony, on the other hand, can bear a few sleepless nights and function as normal for the most part. But that would mean we would need Taj to be on the bottle in order for D'Anthony to wake up at night and give Rachel the time she needs to sleep and function. We worked it out—a good example of one of the ways we have found to balance each other out. It may not seem like much, but it still provided relief for Rachel.

The more you're able to identify your strengths and vulnerabilities in the relationship, the more effectively you'll be able to account for them and accomplish tasks together. And that teamwork makes life go much smoother.

In His Words

For some reason, I'm awful at logging on to websites and paying bills. It takes too much focus—maybe it's the repetitiveness that I find so challenging. Rachel, on the other hand, can pay bills while playing with Taj and Aaliyah, while she's in the middle of cooking dinner, all while watching her favorite Netflix show. It goes without saying that Rachel is solely responsible for paying the bills in our house. The fact that we were able to identify this early allowed us to bypass issues that may have come up if we had gotten stuck relying on me to struggle through this particular task.

CONSIDERATIONS AND EXPECTATIONS

The goal for this month is to revisit your shared values and align on what you want the birthing experience to look like. Ideally, you've begun or even completed birthing classes. These classes will help you understand what aspects of the birthing process will require decision-making, and how you can work together to devise a plan around your shared values and respective strengths.

Birth Preference and Plans

Your "birth preferences" are the things that you prefer to happen in a specific way. Your birth plan is just the communication of those preferences, which you can put in writing and share with your birthing team (OB-GYN, midwife, doula, partner, and/or any family or friends who may be present).

However, let us tell you, the most stressful thing you can do to yourself is expect for your plan to go exactly the way you want. It may all work out according to plan, but nature's a funny thing. The best mindset for birth is being educated yet open to changes and making decisions as you go. This is one reason that establishing your shared values prior to the birth is so important. Giving birth takes a lot of energy, so the non-birthing partner should be prepared to take on decision-making if needed during the birth. Getting in sync with each other's preferences will help with this.

In Her Words

I am a type-A planner, so of course I had a plan for Taj's birth: I'd have a vaginal delivery with an epidural; my OB would deliver the baby, followed by immediate skin-to-skin contact and breastfeeding; we'd play my gospel music playlist while D'Anthony, my mom, and my sister supported me the entire time. Fast-forward to the end of the story: Taj was over a week late, and I had to be induced and ended up having a C-section. I didn't play any gospel music, and I learned that three people was too many to have in the room. I did get an epidural, my OB did deliver, and I got to enjoy skin-to-skin contact and breast-feed our new baby. Moral of the story: Know your preferences, but be flexible!

Here are some preferences you may want to consider:

- Birthing location: home, birthing center, or hospital

- Birthing team: OB, doula, or midwife

- Who will be present in the delivery room? In the waiting room?

- Atmosphere/vibe: music, aromatherapy (no flames), crystals

- Pain management: epidural, acetaminophen, no medication

- Nursing or bottle feeding

- Can/will the baby leave the room for any testing (vision, hearing, blood tests)?

- For boys: Will he be circumcised?

- After delivery, who can visit at the hospital and who can visit once you're home? (More on this later.)

Spiritual and Cultural Considerations

Part of the advance planning for the arrival of your new baby may include spiritual or cultural ceremonies. Depending on your individual and shared values, cultures and spiritual beliefs, you may want to discuss the possibility of including traditions that serve an important role in your life. Some common traditions include a bris, baptism, christening, or other introduction into a community, as well as circumcision, ear piercing, burying the placenta, and naming ceremonies, to name a few. Some spiritual traditions require advance planning, such as attendance at classes, so consider using this time to find out more about those requirements.

Baby Shower

Baby showers give loved ones the opportunity to celebrate the pregnant couple and their new addition and see the pregnant person, and, of course, to offer gifts of baby items to help the couple in their new journey. This event can be anything from an intimate couples gathering to a family barbecue to a lavish restaurant affair, depending on your preferences and your circle of family and friends. If you have a large family and friends spread across multiple states, you may find yourselves the guests of honor at multiple showers.

The host is usually a family member or close friend of the pregnant person. This person will be responsible for planning the entire event, from invitations to venue, food, and games.

In Her Words

We worked together to choose the shower host, location, and timing. We wanted to select someone to host whom we could count on as responsible, organized, and friendly. Choosing one's own shower host might sound uncustomary, but it worked for us! My sister and D'Anthony's mother collaborated on our Cleveland shower, and the shower in Connecticut was hosted by my close friend.

The best time for a shower is during the third trimester, if for no other reason than to maximize the cuteness of the bump for photo ops and games. Just don't veer too close to the due date, as you don't want to miss your own shower because you went into labor early! You'll also want time to assess what items from your registry you still need to purchase after the shower.

If your shower isn't a surprise, you can create an invite list and share with the host. Don't be shy about inviting people! Even if you know they can't make it, people like to feel included. Our showers were both coed, which seems to be the norm for the millennial generation and younger, but it's really a personal decision.

For us, both of our families live in the same city, but we live in a different state, and our friends are spread out across numerous states, as well. For Taj, we had two showers: one in Cleveland, Ohio, for family and childhood friends, and one in Connecticut, where we lived at the time, for friends. Rachel's coworkers also threw her a shower at work. Even with Aaliyah, who was born during the COVID pandemic, we had two virtual showers: one for family and one for friends.

If you're having a shower out of town, consider how you'll get the gifts back home. A few options could include driving if it's feasible, so you can just pack up the car and go; requesting all gifts be shipped to your home instead of given in person; or shipping all the gifts after the shower—by far the costliest option.

Regardless of whether your shower is in-person or virtual, this is one of those memorable moments in the journey worth capturing. For the pregnant person, prepare in whatever way makes you feel good. If you like, get your hair, makeup, and/or nails done, and find something stylish to wear that accentuates your belly.

After the baby shower, cross-check the gifts you received against your registry list and determine what remaining items you still really need. Take stock of the clothes that were purchased, organizing them by size. Unless you deliver prematurely, you generally won't need a lot of newborn clothes, since you're likely not going too many places for the first six weeks other than the doctor's. We had a week's worth of onesies and pajamas (about 10–15 onesies and 4–5 jammies should do the trick) and just washed those as needed. In terms of clothes, we made sure to have the bulk of items for 0 to 6 months and didn't buy anything extra beyond those sizes initially.

Controlling Your Own Gate

It's important to clearly communicate to family and friends your guidelines for visiting the baby and when. How you plan for this might be one of your most important check-ins as a couple. Before your baby comes, we recommend sitting down and deciding together:

WHO YOU WANT (AND DON'T WANT) TO VISIT IN THE HOSPITAL. Hospital rules vary: Some hospitals allow 24/7 visitors; others will restrict visitors to one person at a time. The more liberal visiting hours may seem enticing *until* your well-meaning friend comes by with her two rowdy kids and doesn't know when to take a hint that you're tired. Choose your visitors in advance, and feel free to be clear on your limitations.

WHO YOU WANT (AND DON'T WANT) TO VISIT YOUR HOME AFTER THE BABY COMES HOME. We'll discuss this more later, but it's good to start the conversation now. Who do you want to visit? Who are you not ready for? What hours will work for visitors?

WHAT BOUNDARIES YOU'LL SET. They say that nobody can violate your boundaries without your permission. It's so important for your well-being and recovery to maintain strong boundaries during this time. Just because a friend calls does not mean you have to answer. If someone shows up at your door, you do not need to let them in. Decide how you will address these conversations. You may need to practice your assertiveness so you can say, "Thanks for thinking of us, but we're not up to visitors today. I'll let you know when we're feeling up to it."

WHAT STRATEGIES YOU'LL USE. Being in tune with each other is key here. Non-birthing partner, if you have guests and see your partner looks tired, your heroic deed can be to tell your guests that visiting time is over and your partner needs rest: "C'mon, I'll walk you to the door." Emo deposit! For the partner who just gave birth, when you've had enough, it's okay to interrupt somebody mid-sentence and say, "I have to go rest now." Let your body language do the talking. Lie back and close your eyes. They will get the clue.

Hot-Button Issues Like Vaccinations and Circumcision

Several big decisions need to be made as a team, including a couple that have the potential to stir up controversy, both within your household and even beyond. Different communities feel strongly regarding practices like vaccinations and circumcisions. The important question, though: Where do you stand?

A great place to start these discussions is by sharing your individual feelings on the matter. If you're not in clear alignment, revisit your family values and consider whether you feel that the procedures you're discussing are in alignment with those values. Generally, it is assumed by medical providers that vaccinations will be given. You might be asked if you want to have your baby circumcised, but it's possible they will just assume you are having it done. If, however, you're in agreement that you don't want your baby vaccinated and/or circumcised, give your admitting hospital and pediatrician advance notice that you would like to bypass these procedures.

Whether you choose to vaccinate or circumcise or not, be sure to learn about any associated risks or side effects of doing so or not doing so. If you bypass these procedures, find out about the alternatives to these methods, the time they may take to implement, and any additional paperwork needed. For example, there is generally paperwork needed surrounding vaccinations when a child is enrolled in childcare or school.

You'll also want to carefully consider who will be around your child, particularly in the first six weeks, before they receive key immunizations and while their immune systems are developing. Normal guidance is for newborns to steer clear of any unvaccinated persons (including COVID), especially in the first six weeks, and to be around only those who are up-to-date with their DTAP vaccination. Depending on your family values, this guidance could affect who visits or provides support immediately following birth.

DIVIDE AND CONQUER

This month, take time to enjoy each other and your family and friends. The shift to the third trimester will start to weigh more heavily on the pregnant person, both figuratively and literally. The non-birthing partner will need to help in different ways during these final months, while the pregnant person will need to speak up as needed so the non-birthing partner knows how they can best help.

TIME-SENSITIVE

- Baby shower

- Babymoon

RESEARCH AND DISCUSS

- Birth preferences for birth plan

- Spiritual or cultural traditions

- Weekly baby development video (see Resources, page 172)

SCHEDULE AND PLAN

- Maternity or baby bump photo shoot

- Couple check-in

ADDITIONAL

_____

_____

_____

_____

_____

_____

_____

_____

_____

_____

_____

_____

_____

DECIDE TOGETHER

Use these sheets to help you get on the same page when you're facing a tricky decision, like choosing a name or figuring out childcare.

YOUR PROBLEM OR DESIRED GOAL: _____

_____

What's important to Partner A?	What's important to Partner B?

Circle the top one to three things that matter most to you. Take turns explaining to your partner why your circled items are important to you. Then take some time separately to research and brainstorm solutions. List all your ideas, even wild or unusual ones.

_____

_____

_____

_____

_____

_____

List any factors that will impact your decision. This is where you set reasonable boundaries (time, cost, effort, etc.) about your possible solutions.

_____

_____

_____

_____

_____

_____

_____

_____

Partner A's short list	Partner B's short list

Discuss which solution is best for your relationship. Can you come to an enthusiastic agreement?

OUR FINAL DECISION: _____

Nesting and Documenting

This month, as you inch closer to the birth of your baby, you'll be preparing your home for your new addition and starting to consider the routines that come along with parenthood. You don't need to focus so much about the routines themselves, because you'll undoubtedly figure out what works for you without our help. We're here to talk you through the pros and the cons of establishing these routines and how they can affect life with your partner.

WHAT'S PHYSICALLY HAPPENING

During month eight, the pregnant partner's mood may start to shift from pregnancy joy or normalcy to pregnancy annoyance. Somewhere between this month and next month, they may start to feel ready to deliver and be done with pregnancy. This is also the month to stop traveling long distances from home, whether by air or car, and stay within a reasonable distance to home in case of early labor. This doesn't mean that you can't go out and enjoy a night on the town; by all means, celebrate! While pregnant with Taj, we attended a winter gala an hour from home, and enjoyed a night of music, food, and hanging out with friends. It felt great.

At this point, both partners should continue to monitor how different activities affect the energy level of the pregnant person and plan accordingly. The gala we attended was from 6:00 p.m. until midnight, so we booked a hotel for the night and arrived early so that Rachel could take a nap before the event started. You may start to feel more tired as delivery gets closer, so take advantage of naps whenever you can.

The baby is typically quite active in this month, which may cause increased discomfort for the pregnant person. This could include more trips to the bathroom because of the increasing size and weight of the baby on your bladder. You may experience swollen feet, and perhaps some back or pelvic pain due to increased weight or positioning of the baby. It can also be difficult finding a comfortable sleeping position. Non-birthing partner, more heroic emo deposits you can offer include foot or lower back massages, helping prop pillows, tying shoes, or even running out for ice cream late at night. These kinds of tender gestures will be long remembered.

Your baby is developing quickly now, gaining more weight and increased brain and lung development, as well as improving in their eyesight and hearing. By the end of this month, your baby will be about the size of a honeydew melon. All of this growth is often accompanied by strong movement, and you may even notice a pattern. Some babies may be more active at night, which can interfere with sleep. Rubbing the belly near the baby, talking, singing, or playing music can all be helpful tools for soothing and calming the baby and parent. These are tactics that both partners can utilize, and sometimes solidarity from the non-birthing partner is all the pregnant person needs. If you can afford to miss a couple of hours of sleep, maybe you can stay up with your partner and just keep them company.

TEAM TOOLBOX

This Month's Strategy: Routines: Pros, Cons, and Tips

When we build a life with someone, we begin to develop certain routines. Routines are great because they save us time and valuable brain capacity, and they allow us to essentially act without much effort or thought. In the future, your baby will generally eat at a certain time every day, take naps at the same time every day, and go to sleep at about the same time every day. And if your baby is on a routine, you'll also have a routine. Maybe you'll use nap time to fold clothes, prepare dinner, or work on some business-related task. These are all very productive things that need to be done; however, too much of a routine can open you up to monotony and rigidity, two archenemies of a vibrant, evolving relationship. While we know these routines help make household tasks organized and predictable, when it comes to you and your partner, consider making a promise to use some of your downtime together. That time can be spent watching TV, chopping veggies together, or just sitting on the porch and having an adult conversation—bonus points if you don't talk about your kids!

It's easy to think that your time is best spent cleaning or folding clothes while your baby is sleeping, but putting your relationship first comes with a long-term incentive that can't be outdone by clean floors. Start implementing this strategy now so it becomes muscle memory later: Every day, set aside time for your relationship. Do anything you want; just be present with each other, without phones or distractions.

And when your beautiful baby comes and takes over your world, use this strategy to ensure that you continue to remember, honor, and celebrate the importance of Team You.

CONSIDERATIONS AND EXPECTATIONS

This month is all about preparing for your baby to come home. You've been anticipating and visualizing this moment for months, so before it becomes reality, take some time to outline what else needs to be done to be ready for baby to come home. Avoid procrastinating, because if you happen to go into early labor, you don't want to realize that no one bought the car seat or come home and have to put together a crib. With good humor, let's call this "the calm before the storm"—the ideal time to get organized and take care of anything left to be done.

Nesting

Nesting is the sudden urge to prepare your home for your baby's arrival. While you may have your own agenda, here are some suggestions to get organized:

- Decorate the nursery.

- Sterilize/wash bottles (even if you plan on nursing, it's good to have a few just in case).

- Wash, fold, and organize the baby's clothes, bedding, and blankets.

- Set up the nursery, assemble the crib and furniture, decorate the room, set up and test the baby monitor, rearrange your bedroom if you plan to use a bassinet or co-sleeper.

- Prepare for any feeding needs (formula, nursing bras, pads, etc.) if needed.

- Stock up on sanitary pads for after childbirth (the hospital may give you supplies for this).

This nesting may also spill over to the house in general, as you clean and organize around the house to make space for your new baby and their gear.

Finalizing Postpartum Supports

If you haven't finalized them, these preparations should also include some last-minute planning for postpartum care and support. The shift from no children to a child is a huge leap. The first several weeks come with a big learning curve, so having supports in place for that initial time frame is a game changer.

For both pregnancies, Rachel used a mix of parental leave, personal time, sick time, and vacation time to cover her leave—she took 16 consecutive weeks off with Taj and 18 weeks off with Aaliyah. D'Anthony had four weeks of parental leave that could be taken in one-week increments, so both times we opted for him take his first week off as soon as the baby was born in order to have uninterrupted bonding time and support Rachel. (This postpartum support is especially important after a C-section.) He then waited to take his remaining three weeks until after Rachel returned to work to stretch out the time before the baby would need to enter someone else's care.

Beyond yourselves, consider outside help for two time frames: the first few weeks after you come home, and after you return to work, if applicable. Those first weeks are life-changing. You have a whole brand-spanking-new human to figure out and take care of around the clock. It's easy to forget about yourselves and the care and nourishment that each of you also need, because you will be consumed with ensuring that your baby is perfectly content.

Some factors to consider are meals, rest, and self-care. Having an extra person around, whether on a daily basis or to drop by every day for a few hours, will help free up time for you new parents to eat, take a nap, or enjoy a shower that lasts more than two minutes. Consider if you have any retired family and friends or someone who has a flexible work schedule or is willing to take vacation days to come help. Key to this is ensuring that whomever you select will provide relief and not increase stress in the household.

Even if you don't have someone who can come stay with you, having nearby friends or family come over to bring a meal or some groceries, do a load of laundry, clean up, or even watch the baby while you nap is a gift you'll not soon forget.

The final piece of the postpartum care puzzle is formal childcare. Hopefully you've decided on a childcare approach to start with, but it's okay to be flexible. Don't be afraid to make a change if it's not working for you. The first day care that we tried for Taj was discounted through our job (we both worked for the same parent company); plus, many parents we worked with had their children there, and it was within walking distance of our work office. However, after a couple of months, we felt that there were too many babies in the class and Taj wasn't getting as much focused attention as we would have liked. So we found another day care through a coworker's recommendation. It was more expensive and a little farther away, but we felt the care was better. We decided to switch him, and we were so happy with the move that we kept him there until we relocated.

Documenting

Throughout this book, we've suggested you capture special moments like the first ultrasound, gender reveal, babymoon, and baby shower with pictures or videos, as well as the everyday moments, whether you're on walks together, cooking dinner, or just sitting on the couch. Rachel took a weekly picture of her belly to document the growth. Sometimes it's hard to remember to capture the moments while you're living them, but if you haven't taken the time yet, don't panic! This is your best opportunity of all: a maternity or baby bump photo shoot!

This photo shoot can be as grand or as low-key as you want it to be. Documenting these special moments will provide fun memories and cute pictures, but even more, the photo shoot is a moment that is just about you, your partner, and your baby-to-be. With Taj, we went the low-key route. We wore blue jeans and we asked a photographer friend to come to our house to take pictures inside and on the deck. D'Anthony is pretty good with a camera, so he added to our maternity shoot by taking portraits of Rachel in the nursery and living room.

With Aaliyah, we went a bit bigger. We enlisted a photographer with a studio, and Rachel brought two outfits: an elaborate maternity gown we ordered from Mama Bump Rentals (see Resources, page 173) and a floor-length tulle skirt and cropped blouse. We even asked one of Rachel's best friends to serve as our stylist, picking coordinating outfits for D'Anthony and Taj. The photo shoot took almost four hours, including makeup, two wardrobe changes, and the photo session. The pictures came out great and it was worth it, but if you go this route, just make sure you're prepared with food, drinks, and time to rest in between shots.

In Her Words

Christmas also occurred in this month while we were pregnant with Taj. There are so many creative ways to celebrate a holiday with a baby on the way: I bought a miniature stocking and hung it on the fireplace along with ours and surprised D'Anthony by getting a personalized bracelet with Taj's name on it—my way of telling him that I agreed to the name he picked.

DIVIDE AND CONQUER

This is the month to research, get recommendations from family and friends, and document the process of the home stretch. If possible, schedule a tour of the birthing center where you plan to deliver—this is sometimes included with birthing classes, but it varies by facility. Revisit your shared values and how they will translate during childbirth and after the baby has arrived. Partners, continue to lean in and support each other as much as you can these last two months.

TIME-SENSITIVE

- Nursery setup
- Maternity or baby bump photo shoot

RESEARCH AND DISCUSS

- Postpartum care and support
- Names
- Weekly baby development video (see Resources, page 172)

SCHEDULE AND PLAN

- Birthing center/labor and delivery tour
- Birth plan
- Couple check-in

ADDITIONAL

_____

_____

_____

_____

_____

_____

_____

_____

_____

_____

_____

_____

_____

Advocate, Advocate, Advocate

In 2020, the Centers for Disease Control and Prevention (CDC) released a report noting that the US maternal mortality rate has risen, even as worldwide mortality rates have dropped. Frighteningly, the maternal mortality rate is nearly three times higher for Black women. As members of the Black community, we were aware of this. We'd heard stories of denied pain medicine requests or complaints about dismissed symptoms, sometimes a more serious issue being missed.

Our friend Charles Johnson started a nonprofit, 4Kira4Moms (see Resources, page 173), which advocates for improved maternal health policies and regulations in the United States, educates the public about the Black maternal mortality crisis, supports families and friends impacted directly by this crisis, and promotes the idea that maternal mortality is a human rights issue. It also lobbies for legislation that requires sensitivity and bias training for medical staff.

The statistics and stories about maternal mortality rates can be frightening, regardless of your background or identity, but for families from historically marginalized communities, there may be a heightened level of anxiety. That's why it's important for couples to discuss and agree on a birth plan in advance, and for the non-birthing partner to be present, involved, and vocal leading up to and during the delivery. The pregnant partner will need your support and advocacy on their behalf.

When the time comes, don't be afraid to ask clarifying questions, pushing if needed until you have very clear and direct answers. For example, if a C-section is recommended by your doctor because you aren't progressing as quickly as they would like, ask, "What are my options?" and "What are the risks if we decline?" Keep an eye on your partner's level of awareness, body language, and vocalizations, and involve them in decisions whenever possible. If there is a nurse or birth team member who is not respecting your wishes, ask the head nurse on call to replace them. It can also help to talk to friends who've already experienced childbirth for advice on how they advocated for themselves, too.

DECIDE TOGETHER

Use these sheets to help you get on the same page when you're facing a tricky decision, like choosing a name or figuring out childcare.

YOUR PROBLEM OR DESIRED GOAL: _____

_____

What's important to Partner A?	What's important to Partner B?

Circle the top one to three things that matter most to you. Take turns explaining to your partner why your circled items are important to you. Then take some time separately to research and brainstorm solutions. List all your ideas, even wild or unusual ones.

_____

_____

_____

_____

_____

_____

List any factors that will impact your decision. This is where you set reasonable boundaries (time, cost, effort, etc.) about your possible solutions.

_____

_____

_____

_____

_____

_____

_____

Partner A's short list	Partner B's short list

Discuss which solution is best for your relationship. Can you come to an enthusiastic agreement?

OUR FINAL DECISION: _____

Last-Minute Preparations

You've made it to the home stretch! This month is about finishing the last layer of preparations as you transition into childbirth and your new experience of living together with your child. There are some practical things we can do this month that will make things a bit easier. With this new transition may come some feelings you weren't expecting. We'll discuss how to give yourself and your partner "permission to grow" during this pivotal time in your relationship.

WHAT'S PHYSICALLY HAPPENING

For the pregnant partner, your belly is likely quite large, heavy, and taxing on your body, particularly your back and pelvis. You may feel tired and not be able to sleep well (or sleeping in awkward positions) due to the challenge of trying to find a comfortable position.

In His Words

On the upside, you may be eating everything in sight and have a go-to favorite snack or meal. I say, have your fun where you can! While Rachel was pregnant with Aaliyah, she enjoyed a McDonald's M&M's McFlurry almost every night during the weeks leading up to the due date.

Your baby is developed enough to deliver at any time. A full-term baby is generally the size of a watermelon, so you may start to notice less movement because they don't have as much space, and you will likely start to experience more discomfort in your pelvic area as the baby starts to drop down into delivery position.

TEAM TOOLBOX

This Month's Strategy: Give Each Other Grace

In a relationship, it's very easy to set expectations. Our expectations are influenced by our childhood and life experiences, as well as the ideas and people we're exposed to. Based on your family experiences, you may have a very specific idea of what role your partner will play in raising your child. These expectations tend to become more obvious as a relationship progresses. Whether your relationship is on the newer side or you've been in a relationship for years, it's safe to assume that you and your partner will both undergo an evolution of some kind while you're together. Your respective views on some subjects may change over the years, or they may stay the same (sometimes for longer than you would hope).

Whatever the situation, it's very important to give each other both time and space to grow and evolve. For example, when we first met, Rachel expected D'Anthony to be able to fully understand her feelings right away when she brought up things that bothered her. Similarly, D'Anthony expected Rachel to be able to change her behavior immediately if something she did bothered him. But getting to know a person takes time, and so does adjusting the expectations that come with that. Knowing this, we tried to give each other grace, which made it easier to stay patient when one of us did something to disappoint the other.

Changing your expectations for a person is easier said than done; you may be wondering how to do this. For us, it comes back to our shared values, which are empathy, respect, autonomy, and trust. Empathy helps us see that when someone's acting out of character, it may be because they're not feeling right inside. Under their annoying or triggering behavior, there might be tough feelings due to past experiences or old beliefs. We also try to treat each other with respect, even when we're feeling furious or overwhelmed, so no one is feeling shamed or attacked during conflicts. We remind ourselves that our partner has autonomy over their choices, which means we see that we can't force a person to do something that they are not ready to do. And in the end, we fall back on trust and the knowledge that no matter what, we're always trying to do our best with the resources we have available to us at that time.

Giving each other room to grow gives you both permission to think freely and change without being penalized, and being able to think freely allows you to grow on your own terms, avoid resentment, and ultimately become a more cohesive and effective team.

CONSIDERATIONS AND EXPECTATIONS

These last few weeks will include more frequent visits to the doctor, and a couple of new tests. The pregnant partner will be tested for Group B Strep, a bacteria that could be passed to the baby during delivery and cause an infection. The doctor will send a vaginal swab for testing. If it comes back positive, it's nothing to panic over. Discuss your treatment plan with your doctor—it will likely include giving you antibiotics during the labor process, which will stop you from passing the bacteria to the baby.

Your cervix and the baby's position will be checked each visit. The cervix check is to determine if you are dilating or effacing, either of which would mean you're getting close to starting labor. The doctor will also check that the baby's position is head down. If the baby is facing head up, the doctor may offer guidance for getting the baby to flip or suggest a procedure. This is something the pregnant person and partner will need to decide on together. If the baby doesn't flip to head-down position, the doctor will ultimately schedule a C-section, as it is generally not safe to deliver vaginally when the baby is head up.

At this time, you can go into labor at any point, so be prepared and keep your phones handy. Think about things like having the overnight bag packed for your stay at the delivery center, keeping the car's gas tank filled, and making sure all the preparations are complete at home. Accept that you may not remember everything. Just do one final sweep and then relax.

Beyond that, the goal for this month is to rest and be confident that you've done everything you can to prepare for the arrival of your child. Go out to a nice dinner if you feel like it, catch a movie, invite friends over for a game night. After all your preparation, you deserve to unwind and do something fun together.

Creating a Healthy Support System

When it comes to support systems, think about the people in your community who know how to support you. There may be many wonderful people who love you and want to help, but not everyone will know how to support you during every season of your life. Learning to manage those relationships can be hard.

For us, we've found that being direct with the people who don't support us in the way we need to be supported is the best approach. If there's a family member who likes to come over and spend time with you during your pregnancy, that is a kind gesture, but it may not fit your current need. And it can seem uncomfortable to just dismiss them. Try using clear communication, like "Today's not a good day for me. Can I let you know when it's a good time to come over?" Sentences that explicitly put the ball in your court are always the most clear. Try to stay away from sentences like "You don't have to do that" or "I don't want to take time away from you," which are generally seen as a kind decline and left open for interpretation. This diplomatic work can be handled by either partner.

Sometimes close friends, especially ones who already have kids, can be the most supportive. Shortly after Taj was born, one of our close couple friends brought their kids over and told us to leave and that they would watch Taj while we got dinner. This was our first time out of the house together without Taj.

If you're pregnant for the first time, finding other pregnant couples can be great. Sometimes you just need one person who knows what you're experiencing—from the pregnant person perspective and the non-birthing partner perspective. As previously mentioned, we were pregnant with Taj at the same time as three other couples that we were good friends with. The best part of this came after all the babies were born, when we automatically had a little group for babysitting exchanges, playdates, and birthday parties!

DIVIDE AND CONQUER

Your baby is coming to town, and this time it's you who needs to make a list and check it twice. At this point, the only things that matter are what you and the baby will need to leave the hospital, come home, and make it through the first week. Everything else can be figured out or purchased later. Don't forget, these are your last few weeks as a party of two!

TIME-SENSITIVE

- Install car seat

- Download a contraction timer app (see Resources, page 172)

- Decide on a name (or a short-list of names)

- Pack hospital bags for the pregnant person (and the non-birthing partner if needed)

RESEARCH AND DISCUSS

- Family/friend communication plan during delivery

- Weekly baby development video (see Resources, page 172)

SCHEDULE AND PLAN

- Date night

- Couple check-in

ADDITIONAL

_____

_____

_____

_____

_____

_____

_____

_____

_____

_____

_____

_____

_____

_____

_____

_____

_____

_____

_____

_____

_____

_____

_____

DECIDE TOGETHER

Use these sheets to help you get on the same page when you're facing a tricky decision, like choosing a name or figuring out childcare.

YOUR PROBLEM OR DESIRED GOAL: _____

_____

What's important to Partner A?	What's important to Partner B?

Circle the top one to three things that matter most to you. Take turns explaining to your partner why your circled items are important to you. Then take some time separately to research and brainstorm solutions. List all your ideas, even wild or unusual ones.

_____

_____

_____

_____

_____

_____

_____

List any factors that will impact your decision. This is where you set reasonable boundaries (time, cost, effort, etc.) about your possible solutions.

_____

_____

_____

_____

_____

_____

_____

_____

Partner A's short list	Partner B's short list

Discuss which solution is best for your relationship. Can you come to an enthusiastic agreement?

OUR FINAL DECISION: _____

PART FOUR

BIRTH AND BEYOND

Labor and Delivery

This is the day that all your preparations collide with the unique and privileged childbirth experience. The two of you know your roles perfectly—you're an awesome team—and for the non-birthing partner, all that you've learned has prepared you to keep your partner feeling motivated and encouraged. You've both totally got this.

WHAT'S PHYSICALLY HAPPENING

This is it: Your baby is coming, either vaginally or via C-section. That said, the vaginal birth process has no specific timeline. Yes, you have a due date, but the baby may come early, late, or on time. Vaginal birth consists of three stages: (1) early and active labor, (2) delivery of the baby, and (3) delivery of the placenta. This type of delivery can be performed at home, a birthing center, or a hospital. For a vaginal birth in the hospital, you will likely spend a good amount of time at home having contractions before you go to the hospital to deliver.

A C-section involves surgery in an operating room. You would receive spinal anesthesia to numb the body, leaving you fully awake for the procedure but unable to feel anything. The C-section birth process can be planned or unplanned. Planned C-sections occur when there is some predetermined reason, such as that the baby is not positioned head down, or other specific concerns preventing you from delivering the baby vaginally. In this case, you'll schedule a C-section at the hospital on a specific date at a specific time. An unplanned C-section means your plan A was a vaginal delivery but complications arose. Perhaps the cervix is not dilating or effacing, the baby is in distress, or you are in distress. A C-section tends to be a much faster delivery, enabling medical personnel to respond to any of the baby's or mother's needs more quickly.

TEAM TOOLBOX

This Month's Strategy: An Unbreakable Team

Pregnancy is a team sport. At the beginning of this book, we spoke about the non-birthing partner's role and how they could support, while allowing their pregnant partner to do the things they felt up to doing. You've done a great job. Now that the birth is nearly upon you, your role becomes that of the dependable rock: staying cool, levelheaded, and present as you make your partner feel comfortable in every way possible. Your head may be spinning—that's normal. You've got this—all the check-ins, emo deposits, and honest communication have brought your relationship to a deeper level of understanding and preparedness.

For both of you, this entire book boils down to being effective partners. It's about communication, understanding your partner's needs and wants, and figuring out a way to balance them with your own. Even as you become parents, agreeing on the roles each of you will play while making sure those are the roles that come most naturally to you will be key to a healthy and fulfilled relationship. And this can evolve. You may find over time that one of you becomes more involved in a certain area, and that's good too, as long as you're communicating. When you're in agreement about what each person brings to the table, you'll cultivate a strong and enduring bond with no resentment.

Imagine everything that you and your partner have been through. Recall the intentional steps you each took to ensure that the other felt seen and understood. If you've been reading this book, that means you've been participating in these very positive intentional actions for the past nine months. At this point, showing love and intentionality toward each other is no longer a calculated practice—it has now graduated to a lifestyle.

EARLY LABOR

This is where things get exciting. Early labor means your body is beginning its preparation for delivery. During this process, your cervix is dilating (opening) and effacing (softening and thinning) in order for the baby to pass through. The time frame for this varies greatly, from a few hours to several days.

What are signs of early labor?

You will begin to feel contractions, or tightness and hardening, in your belly; you may also feel it in your back. This is generally the longest part of labor and delivery, and depending on your proximity to the hospital or birthing center, you'll generally want to stay home for as long as possible before going to the hospital (unless you've been directed otherwise). If you do go to the hospital before your body is ready to go into active labor, you may be sent home to wait longer.

Other common signs of early labor are bleeding that may look similar to your menstrual cycle bleed, commonly referred to as the bloody show; the water breaking, which is the amniotic sac that housed the baby for all these months; and the release of a mucus-like discharge, which is the mucus plug.

Feel free to reach out to your medical provider with an update. Let them know if your water broke. If you're concerned about anything you're feeling or seeing, it's best to call. Many OB-GYNs have a labor hotline or after-hours receptionist, who can route you to an on-call nurse or doctor for guidance. If you have a doula or midwife, now is the time to reach out to them, as well.

How do we know when it's time to go to the hospital?

For most people, the gold standard for when to go to the hospital for delivery is the 5-1-1 rule. You may have learned this in your birthing class. 5-1-1 stands for:

- Contractions that occur every 5 minutes,

- last for 1 minute each,

- and have been happening consistently for at least 1 hour.

Non-birthing partners, you're the timekeeper. Simply monitor the time using an app (see Resources, page 174) or a watch or phone (and write it down), so your partner can focus on breathing and staying as calm as possible.

When your water breaks, call your doctor, doula, or midwife and let them decide whether you should go in. If you have excessive bleeding, unbearable pain, or anything that just doesn't seem right, the safe thing to do is head to the hospital and call your doctor on the way.

What can partners do to help the laboring pregnant person?

The key to success for this stage is to stay calm. You can even try to keep busy together. Try to focus on breathing and the exercises you learned during the birthing classes. Partners, lean in and encourage relaxation. Go on a walk together, run a bath, play some music, and/or help with stretching or massage. Even though partners may not be able to eliminate discomfort, being actively involved in each stage will help and enhance the experience for both of you.

An important part of labor not often discussed is keeping the baby calm. Labor can be a stressful event for both the pregnant person and the baby, and the pregnant person's stress could affect the baby's stress levels, potentially causing the baby's heart rate to rise to an unsafe level. You can help by rubbing the belly, talking to the baby, or playing music. Most of all, always trust your intuition. The pregnant person may be saying everything is okay, but if something doesn't look or sound right to you, call the doctor.

What if you don't go into labor?

So, week 40 comes and goes, and you're still sitting at home, eating ice cream; no discomfort, no cramping, no blood, nothing! You're officially late. This is not uncommon, especially with first babies. Most doctors will schedule a nonstress test (NST) during week 40 if you haven't gone into labor yet. During a nonstress test, they will monitor the baby's heart rate, checking to make sure the baby is moving well and the heart rate is within normal range. As long as everything is within the normal range, they will let you go home and continue to wait to go into labor. Generally, you will not be allowed to go beyond 42 weeks, so the doctor may schedule you to be induced; that is, given intravenous medication to initiate contractions and labor.

With Taj, Rachel had the nonstress test done at 40 weeks, and her OB preemptively scheduled her to be induced at 41 weeks in case she did not go into labor before then. She did not, and her cervix had made no progress in preparing for the baby: no dilating, no softening, no thinning. There were two parts to our induction process:

Part 1: We arrived and checked in to the hospital. A balloon filled with water was inserted into the vagina, which sits on the cervix and jump-starts the process of dilating and effacing. This caused the uterine muscles to contract and gave Rachel her first insight into the feeling of a contraction (eye-opening!). They kept the balloon in for about 12 hours, and during that time Rachel was able to walk around and do everything as she normally would, other than using the bathroom. They had to insert a catheter, so she was peeing into a bag while she had a balloon full of water inside of her. Science really is amazing.

Part 2: The next morning, they removed the balloon and she was three centimeters dilated but not effaced. The doctors hooked her up to an IV and gave her Pitocin, a medication that causes contractions. Not long after the Pitocin started, the contractions started.

ACTIVE LABOR AND PUSHING

Ah, the joys of active labor. 'Tis what all the movies portray! Everyone will have an image of active labor in their head going into it, likely based off some movie you saw that painted labor in its most heavily dramatized and extreme form. In reality, labor can be quick and relatively calm, or long and strenuous, or anywhere in between. Going in as calmly as possible is the best way to approach it.

In active labor, contractions come quickly and consistently, and the pregnant person is usually uncomfortable, unless they've already received an epidural. We would argue that this is the single most important part of the pregnancy because all of your team-building and planning are put into action. The pregnant person will be absorbed by getting through each contraction, and that should be your sole focus.

This means, non-birthing partner, that you are managing everything else while ideally staying calm—a big job. This "everything else" includes supporting your partner in every way: mentally, by talking to them and encouraging them, playing music if it helps, turning the lights off, or opening a window; physically, by massaging or applying pressure to distract from the contractions, offering ice chips, a heating pad, or a cold damp compress for their head; and anything else the pregnant person requests or needs to get through. In addition, you're now in charge of managing interactions with the hospital staff and any family or friends who may be present or asking for updates.

At some point, if the pregnant partner's water has not broken already, it will break or the doctor will break it, which generally leads to more intense contractions.

In His Words

When Rachel's intense contractions started, I took her phone and became responsible for all communications. I decided who to update and when, and she never asked once about the phone until well after the delivery. I also stayed engaged through most of the contractions unless she told me to give her space, letting her squeeze my hands or stare into my eyes. I picked up on her emotional cues just by looking at her.

In Her Words

My way of getting through contractions was by blurring out the background sounds and bearing down on something, so silence was very helpful to me. That's why, as we mentioned earlier, we never played any music from the gospel playlist we created. As we also mentioned, my sister and mom were in the room for Taj's labor. Although I was happy that they and the nurse were cheering me on through the contractions, I didn't want to hear a pin drop when it came time to bear down and push. D'Anthony could see that in my facial expressions, and he helped to quiet the room.

Throughout all this, it will be important for the non-birthing partner to keep the birth preferences/plan front of mind, and it may be helpful to have a printout, since there will be a lot to keep track of in the moment. The non-birthing partner will need to monitor the pregnant person's requests, and ensure the hospital staff is acting on requests in a timely manner. Are there specific positions for pushing the birth partner wants to try? Is the staff pressuring the pregnant person to do something that is causing unnecessary pain? You'll need to step in and advocate on behalf of your partner.

The epidural is an optional numbing medication that reduces the pain of contractions while still allowing for the feeling of pressure, so you can feel and push when it comes time. It's important to know that there is a window of time in which an epidural mut be given; however, the anesthesia staff is generally on call and not just waiting in the hallway for the pregnant person to be ready. For this reason, there may be a delay from the time you ask for the epidural to the time that you get it. Keep this in mind when considering this option so you don't miss the opportunity.

All this responsibility can be overwhelming for the non-birthing partner. Take a moment to calm your own nerves when you see a chance. When your partner is between contractions and resting quietly, step into the bathroom, take some deep breaths, splash water on your face—whatever helps you settle your own emotions.

The directive to "push" generally comes when the cervix is 10 centimeters dilated. This part of the experience can be very intense for the pregnant person, and everyone experiences this differently. This may look like eyes closed and grunting, squeezing tightly on the non-birthing partner's hand or arm, biting the pillow, loud vocalizations, or any number of other options. Really, you'll never know until you get to that point. Non-birthing partners, you'll want to help reinforce the doctor's instructions: push, stop pushing, breathe.

It bears repeating that the birth process doesn't always go as planned, so prepare to adapt if something changes. After being induced, Rachel labored for more than 12 hours with no major progress. Taj's heart rate dropped every time they increased the induction medication,

Pitocin. Rachel's OB recommended a C-section. It was not ideal and not what we had planned for. But because Rachel was tired, the labor wasn't progressing, and Taj was not responding well, we agreed it was the best course of action.

From there, they prepped the operating room. Only one person is allowed in the OR with the pregnant person. D'Anthony was given a pair of scrubs, and the team brought Rachel to the OR to prep her. This included another catheter and a spinal tap, which is a powerful numbing medication. They positioned her on the OR table and hung a sheet vertically across her chest so she couldn't see the operation happening. Once Rachel was prepped, D'Anthony was escorted in and sat in a chair next to her. He could also see the surgery happening.

The preparation for a C-section, planned or unplanned, is more mental than physical. Depending on how you feel about surgery, the prospect of a C-section can be unsettling, if not downright scary. Before the C-section, there is a brief period when the pregnant person is prepped for surgery and the non-birthing partner is asked to wait outside. You'll be fully numbed from the waist down, and your arms will be strapped to the table to ensure no movement during the surgery. It's important to have some calming strategies for yourself while you wait for your partner to be brought into the OR. Some ideas include deep-breathing exercises, visualizations (such as envisioning a specific location that brings you joy), meditation, self-compassion practices (in which you silently acknowledge your suffering and send yourself love), or even singing a calming song in your head.

In Her Words

I was completely unprepared for this feeling of paralysis and not being able to move anything from my chest down. Even though my second C-section (with Aaliyah) was a planned one, that feeling of not being able to move was still scary, and I began to have a panic attack. D'Anthony's support was absolutely critical at this time: squeezing my hand, talking to me, wiping my tears, and encouraging me to take deep breaths; it was all so helpful in calming me down.

Non-birthing partners, even during C-sections, you can continue to advocate for your birth preferences. In this case, even though Rachel was on the operating table when Taj was born, D'Anthony still made sure to put Taj on her chest for skin-to-skin contact as soon as they gave Taj to him.

BIRTH!

Your baby has arrived! Make sure to give these beginning moments the respect they deserve. Soak up the experience. Take pictures and video, which will allow you to look back and remember the powerful feelings that you had in that moment; do whatever will help you keep these moments embedded in your head forever.

In His Words

Once we saw Taj, there was one thing on our mind: connection. We wanted this child who just entered the world to know exactly who we were, and we wanted to elevate the connection we had developed over the past nine months. When I held Taj for the first time, it was awesome—it was the first time I'd held a baby that small. Rachel was still under a lot of anesthesia and wasn't really coherent, but I knew it was still important for them to physically connect, so I laid Taj on her chest and introduced them to each other.

D'Anthony took pictures, video, and wrote notes about how he was feeling. It was easy to see how some things didn't matter so much, like forgetting to put slippers in the hospital bag, or not finding a close enough parking spot. The feelings and memories that you instantly gravitate toward when you revisit those pictures, videos, or memories will be what matters. It was a great reminder for life to not let the small things ever take away from your overall experience.

When Birth Plans Don't Go as Planned

Blasting music, smiles, sweat, and pushing with success. That's how we thought our delivery process was going to be. A fun experience with some discomfort that we were willing to endure. We created a music playlist full of high energy gospel songs that would surely help see us through. We wanted a vaginal birth that was quick and easy—who doesn't?

We heard so many times how underserved Black women and pregnant people are in healthcare, and we wanted to stay away from medical interventions like C-sections if possible. We were committed to this. But when our doctor recommended a C-section—the very thing that we did not want—we looked at each other and knew that we had to make an important choice. Do we stay the course with our well-thought-out birth plan? Or do we take the new information that the doctor has shared and make adjustments based on what our baby needs?

If you find yourselves in a similar situation, try to look at the big picture and determine what seems best for all three of you. Look at all the choices you've made. Why you chose that hospital; why you chose that doctor; all the research you've done beforehand. And ask yourself: Does it feel right? That's what we did when the plans didn't go our way. We had been induced for days, the labor didn't seem rushed by the doctor and staff, we felt cared about, and the recommendation was coming from a doctor with whom we had a good rapport.

Sometimes birth plans change drastically in ways we really don't want. When that happens, just know that it's okay to have deep and complicated feelings, to have both gratitude and joy for the birth of your baby and grief and disappointment for the loss of the birth experience you'd hoped for. Letting yourself feel your feelings instead of minimizing them and talking about your birth experience with people who can listen with empathy helps, too.

The Newborn Stage

It's mind-blowing to consider how so many life-changing experiences can follow so closely to one another. This is an amazing time: finding out you're pregnant, being pregnant, giving birth, and now bringing this new baby into the life you've lived up until this point. In this chapter, we'll walk you through making the transition from the hospital to your home and deal with some of the life-changing adjustments that come along with a new baby.

WHAT'S PHYSICALLY HAPPENING

The first couple of months are a whirlwind for everyone. It's really a "getting to know you" process. For the pregnant partner, a natural bond already exists between you and your baby from their time spent in the womb and hearing your voices and heartbeat, but now your baby is trying to figure out a whole new world. And as they do, you as parents are attempting to interpret your baby's messages. At times, the learning curve can be fuzzy and frustrating for everyone—this is normal and understandable. The key for you, parents, is to rely on the bond that you've built and strengthened, especially over the last nine months.

For your baby, the first three months will include so much growth and development, you'll be amazed at how much changes every day. Initially, they can't hold their head up, their eyes may not focus or track things, and crying and grunting are their only form of verbal communication. But innately, you will feel what works—what satisfies and makes your baby relax—just by watching their face and feeling their body melt into your arms. In the coming weeks and months, they will be lifting their head and chest, gripping your finger, turning toward sounds, following your movements, recognizing and smiling at you, and even cooing to communicate. It's also fascinating to see how their facial features change so rapidly, especially in the first month. We enjoyed several fun "fights" regarding who they resembled most!

The birthing partner will be going through a lot of changes as well. Your physical healing from the delivery could be minimal; a couple of days if you delivered vaginally with no issues, or a few weeks if you had a C-section. If you're breastfeeding or chestfeeding, once your milk comes in, you may experience engorgement, which is enlarged, sore, or painful tissue resulting from milk production that exceeds what the baby can consume right now. Enlist the aid of pumping, heating pads, and massaging, and reach out to a lactation specialist if you need help. Non-birthing partners can even lean in here: When Rachel was in pain from engorgement, D'Anthony would help massage her breasts while she pumped to get the milk out.

Your hormones will also be adjusting from the pregnancy and nursing and trying to restabilize. Your moods may fluctuate (compounded by missed sleep), and you may also experience hot flashes or night sweats. If this becomes an issue, talk with your doctor; just know that it will eventually balance back out.

It's no surprise that having a new baby takes its toll on energy levels. So while you will be mentally and physically exhausted initially, take comfort in the fact that you will eventually find a routine that works. This routine may not involve all the sleep you might want, but by month three, most parents can identify a structure that works for you, allowing you both to take proper care of yourselves as well.

We're giving this final piece of advice its own space, because it is *that* important:

ASK FOR HELP.

One of the biggest new parenting pitfalls is expecting to be able to do it all on your own, or thinking that asking for help means you're not a good parent or you weren't meant to be a good parent. In truth, a good parent ensures that they take care of themself both mentally and physically, so they can provide the best care for their child. Who can you enlist to help? Consider family, friends, and professionals, depending on the topic or issue. As you make your way through these months and years to come, resist the urge to compare yourself to other parents, or your child to other children. Everyone's situation is different, everyone's development is different, everyone's support structure is different. You are doing you, your way. Do what is best for you and your family.

REAL TALK ABOUT THE MONTHS AHEAD

This new life is a result of everything you have experienced and planned for in the past few months—the life adjustments, the planning, the struggles, and the anticipation. For the last nine months, you may have even looked at the delivering of your baby as the destination; however, you are now absorbing that this is only the beginning of a lifetime of experiences to come.

In His Words

After Rachel's C-section with Taj, we had to stay in the hospital for five days. During that time, we had incredible people showing us how to feed Taj, burp him, recognize his hunger cues, and more. They taught me how to change a diaper—my first time changing a diaper! It was great that we could call someone whenever we had a question. But when it was time to go home, I felt nervous. My very words to Rachel when we left the hospital were, "So, they gonna let us just walk out of here with the baby?" I mean, driver's ed was two weeks in high school—surely after having a baby we should be given at least three weeks of supervision.

For whatever reason, the reality of having a child in our home by ourselves was a terrifying thought. We were convinced that we would be calling the hospital three times a day asking to speak with the nurse to answer our newbie questions. As luck had it, Taj was sleeping when we brought him home. We remembered from all the solicited (and unsolicited) advice we received that you are supposed to "sleep when the baby sleeps." So that's what we tried to do; take a quick nap and wake up when Taj woke up. We used our newly acquired swaddling skills and laid Taj in the bassinet, then we both fell into our bed. As we got comfortable and finally rested our heads on our pillows, we heard the loudest, most massive noise we have ever heard in our entire lives. It was Taj. We were delirious, but we had to get up. The amount of effort it took for us to get out from those incredibly comfortable sheets made us realize that this was going to be an interesting couple of months.

It's Game Time

As nervous as we were, questions like *Can we take care of a baby?* and *Can we even mesh well enough to function?* arose, making us double-guess our abilities. We learned in hindsight that everything was fine. And for you, dear reader, everything will also be fine. These are the two main reasons why:

1. Since you've been reading and referring to this book, you have been practicing techniques that will make you both successful. The emo deposits and the splitting of tasks as you divide and conquer, for example, are strategies that put you in the right mindset for parenting together. You two have experienced a lot together, and you have leaned on each other through some very defining moments of life. You're absolutely ready to tackle these experiences together.

2. You have natural instincts. Situations will arise where you may not know why, but you'll know what to do. You'll tune in to what different cries mean, and you'll instinctively know when your partner has had enough and could use some relief. Though we have outlined very practical strategies in this book, trust in your instincts, for they will give you more good information than any reference material can.

Once you've figured out a routine, a certain confidence level will come along with it. But be warned: A side effect that we've seen in our relationship is that once that routine gets established, anything that goes against how certain tasks are completed might be perceived as wrong or inefficient.

In His Words

When Rachel made Taj's formula, she would put in a carefully measured four scoops plus eight ounces of water. I thought this level of precision was unnecessary. When I made Taj's formula … let's just say there was a little more room for error. This drove Rachel up the wall. There are certain things your partner may do with the baby that goes against the way you think is right. As long as your baby is safe and healthy, we both learned, it's okay to allow each other to do things their way, grow, and be their own person—you know, have autonomy. Different doesn't mean wrong.

Postpartum Depression

Postpartum depression (PPD) was not a term that we were familiar with; of course, we'd heard it used before but never really connected with what it means. Our postpartum period after Taj's birth was normal, the usual exhaustion mixed with the learning curve of first-time parents. PPD had never come up in discussions with any of our other first-time parent friends who'd recently delivered, either.

But things were a little different after Aaliyah's birth. We initially assumed that PPD was something that might last for a few weeks, or worst-case scenario, a few months after giving birth. After all, it makes sense that your partner who just gave birth might feel irritated or frustrated—even sadness or anger—by everything that comes along with the experience. But over time, we slowly started to identify and define postpartum depression signs and situations that we saw coming up. Looking back, we figured out that some of the things Rachel had experienced were related to PPD, too, and we wish we had identified the signs earlier. Our experience led us to want to help normalize the experience and let others know that help is available. Here are some things to remember:

- Know that PPD can occur even if everything goes well.

- Know that PPD does not mean you don't love your baby.

- Couples should develop a library of feeling words to use (I am feeling _____).

- Non-birthing partner, don't take anything personally; there's a reason for this, and it's not always about you.

- Acknowledge the term *postpartum depression* in your relationship.

- Non-birthing partner, you can help by motivating your partner to get outside, talk, open up, and get help if needed. Don't let them spend too much time isolating.

- Postpartum depression is absolutely treatable, and nobody should have to suffer in silence.

- Therapy can help. Resources outside of therapy can help. Get help if needed (see Resources, page 174).

- Birthing partners, it's okay to ease your way back into "regular life," but don't isolate yourself—keep connected.

- Tell your partner what you need.

- Your child is a part of your world and you will bond.

- Life gets easier.

- Love and normalcy go a long way. Hug and get outside and do things.

Postpartum depression is definitely not something we thought about until after Aaliyah was born. In our case, Aaliyah's pregnancy and the several months post-birth were extremely stressful for Rachel. She had an allergic reaction to the surgical gel used to clean her belly before the C-section, and it took four weeks to rectify and heal. Aaliyah would not take a bottle, which meant Rachel had to be at her beck and call every moment and could rarely escape to have any time to herself. Combined with an already stressful pregnancy during a global pandemic, the experience of a second C-section, and fluctuating hormones, this experience was quite overwhelming.

In Her Words

It wasn't until after I had moved past it that I even recognized that I had experienced PPD. My close friend delivered one month after me, and she was experiencing postpartum depression. Through discussions with her, I thought, *Wow, I felt the same way. I experienced that, too.* I talked to D'Anthony about it, and he immediately agreed and said he also felt that I had experienced PPD.

Of course, there will be difficult days, potentially both mentally and physically, depending on your recovery process, but any prolonged feeling of sadness, defeat, or disdain toward the baby is a signal that additional support is needed. Although Rachel did not have much disdain toward Aaliyah, she definitely had her share of moments where she was happier away from her than with her. This has nothing to do with the baby—it is all about a mood disorder that affects the mother's ability to bond and appreciate the experience.

It's critical for the non-birthing partner to watch for the signs, as it's much harder to see the signs when you are actively living it every day. Lastly, it's definitely an area Rachel would have benefited speaking with a health professional about. Now that we know this, we say to you: Please don't suffer in silence or resign yourself to the idea that this is to be expected. It's not, and you don't have to live this way. Know that there is help.

TEAM TOOLBOX

This Month's Strategy: Postpartum Survival Tactics

We're sure every parent in the world can look back on their experience as a first-time parent and identify several things that would have made their lives easier if someone had just told them the cheat code before they had to struggle through it! Well, we're about to give out our cheat codes. Keep in mind, every child is different and every family is different, so whatever you try to implement, make sure it aligns with your shared values and all that you've learned about your child so far.

Team Care

FRIENDS. We found success in allowing a small group of very close friends to bring us dinner every so often. This was never an ask by us. Before each of our babies were born, we had conversations with friends about stories of family members and friends providing dinner for the first couple months. Maybe a huge pot of spaghetti one week, or some bite-size burger bites the next from another set of friends. We were strategic and made sure the generous contributions were spaced out so none of the dishes would go bad. It was fantastic, and we were happy to do the same for our friends when their time came.

SLEEPING. So, how realistic is the adage "Sleep when the baby sleeps"? I'm sure you've heard that many times before, and it's a good strategy if you can sleep on command. Our simple strategy was to figure out who can endure less sleep for that day. There were times Rachel just needed to go to sleep, so D'Anthony was on duty to hold down the fort for the night. There were times when the long nights would get to D'Anthony, but then Rachel was energized, having gotten adequate sleep the previous day, and could cover for him.

COUPLE TIME. We had this preconceived notion with our first child that everything was going to be stressful and a hassle. As a result, we avoided taking Taj out in public. We felt it would be more trouble than it was worth; after all, you have to pack diapers, formula, extra clothes, and more. After a couple of weeks of sitting comfortably in the house, we decided to try our luck and take our newborn baby out to lunch with us. We were paranoid that he would start crying, and we'd be in the restaurant where everyone is looking at us, with no way to calm down this crying baby, making a horrible dining experience for everyone involved.

That couldn't have been further from the truth. We packed up our new baby and his bottles and drove to our favorite restaurant, and we ate tacos and had an adult conversation while Taj slept and peacefully enjoyed the change of scenery. It never really occurred to us that babies can also appreciate a change of scenery.

Of course, now that we have a four-year-old and an almost one-year-old, we realize that bringing a four-week-old baby out of the house is much easier and allows for a greater depth of adult conversation than inviting a three- or four-year-old out to dinner with you. Trust us on this one. There is still room for semi-dates to happen between you two with your infant baby around. Take advantage.

BALANCING DUTIES. We operate like a real-life team. A lot of our skills overlap, so at any point, one of us can pick up the slack for the other, depending on the circumstance. This gives us greater flexibility. If Rachel doesn't feel like cleaning the house or feeding the baby, then there's no problem for D'Anthony to take that on, giving her room to rest, and vice versa when he feels that way. It's very important to be agile and in true partnership and develop the skills to make the household function at its best. AKA, everyone should know how to run the wash!

GOING BACK TO WORK. We were very strategic when it came to our return-to-work plans. We were both in a position to have time off for Taj's birth. Rather than taking that time off together, D'Anthony took the first week off for the birth and days following, while Rachel took her entire leave time before returning to work. Once she went back to work, D'Anthony took his remaining leave time. The strategy was to stretch out as much coverage as possible before having to pay for childcare. Once your leave runs out and your child enters childcare, you'll begin to see how valuable your together time is. Perhaps both parents work until 5:00 p.m. or so, then you pick up your baby from day care around 6:00 p.m. From there you enjoy dinner and some playtime, and then it's time to go to bed. It goes fast.

Baby Feeding

Baby feeding can include human milk, formula, or a combination of both. The general recommendation from pregnancy and medical authorities is to nurse, as human milk has the most nutrients in it for newborn children, among other benefits. However, it's a personal choice that comes down to what is feasible and best for your family. While it can be a beautiful experience, nursing can also be time-consuming and overwhelming, and your well-being is just as important as your child's food source. Our plan was to breastfeed both of our children for one year. We didn't make it to one year for either of them, but we were okay with that because we knew we were doing what we could manage at the time. Some feeding tips:

1. Find a lactation specialist if you plan to breastfeed or chestfeed.

2. Schedule feedings. If using bottles, partners can take turns feeding the baby.

3. Think carefully about when to incorporate a bottle. In our case, we think it can sometimes help to offer a bottle early on. This is a controversial statement, as the general guidance is not to incorporate a bottle immediately because it may cause nipple confusion and potentially lead to a nipple preference. But with Taj, we incorporated the bottle within the first couple of weeks and he had no issues going back and forth between bottle and breast. However, with Aaliyah, we waited to try until after the first month to offer a bottle and she refused it. After four months, we enlisted the help of a consultant who offered bottle-feeding support (see Resources, page 174). This was a game changer, which is why asking for help is so important, and having a lactation specialist on call is helpful.

4. Rinse out bottles right after using. You may be delirious and tired, but try to at least quickly rinse out the bottle, even in your bathroom sink. It doesn't have to be a full clean, but this will make your life easier for the next one, especially if it's the last bottle of the night. You don't want the milk to sit overnight and have to scrub it before you can use it again.

5. If you are nursing and pumping, consider investing in a small freezer. Initially you will produce more milk than the baby can consume, and you may need to pump to relieve the overproduction and potential engorgement. Since the baby is not taking that much milk at first, you can freeze the surplus. We didn't realize how quickly frozen human milk piles up and how much space it takes in your freezer.

Baby Sleep

The American Academy of Pediatrics recommends that newborn babies sleep in the same room with their caregivers because it can decrease the risk of SIDS by as much as 50 percent. But room sharing works well on a more practical level, too, as you'll have to get up and feed the baby multiple times throughout the night. So having the baby close to you is a good thing.

In His Words

One night Taj wouldn't go to sleep. My mom, who was staying with us, came in and rocked him to sleep. As I drifted off, something jolted me awake. Not a crying baby but the thought of my mom putting Taj to sleep on his stomach—a big no-no according to the American Academy of Pediatrics (AAP). Their studies about infant mortality and stomach sleep scared the crap out of us. I checked the baby monitor and saw Taj sleeping comfortably on his stomach. I sprinted to his crib and quickly but gently rolled Taj onto his back... which kept him up all night. Meanwhile, my mom, an "old-school Black mom," huffed that her kids (and nieces' and friends' kids) had all slept on their stomachs and turned out just fine.

Co-sleeping is another option, but that is not recommended by the AAP. There are so many cultural and personal differences that can impact your decision as it relates to a sleeping baby. With our second child we were forced to test this out because Aaliyah would not sleep in a bassinet or a crib. We purchased a highly rated DockATot—a bed or "docking station" that comfortably rests between both parents in their bed. To be clear, this is not recommended by the AAP, but for our desperate situation, it worked for us. In the end, it's best to take all the solid advice and experiences you have collected to make an informed decision for yourself.

Baby Care

There we were, on a family outing before Aaliyah was born, just the three of us. Taj was having a horrible time: inconsolably fussy, didn't want to eat, and only wanted to be held. We got in the car to return home. It was a 30-minute ride, and for 25 of those minutes, Taj screamed his head off. Five minutes from home, he finally fell asleep. We slowly got him out of the car seat, took him in the house, then took off his coat and his socks as smoothly as possible. A diaper check determined that there was no poop, but that he had, in fact, peed. Tough decision in front of us: Do we (A) attempt to change the soaking-wet diaper of a sleeping baby, knowing that if we fail he will be up for many more hours and be very cranky? Or do we (B) put him in his bed, knowing that he has peed in his diaper and that he will sit in it for the next hour and a half? After some debate, we went with option B. You may be faced with the same situation one day, and when you are, just know that baby diapers are incredibly absorbent. There are just some things that are not worth waking a sleeping baby for.

In His Words

Speaking of sleeping babies, here's one more cheat code: I've developed a technique that can be used on any newborn as a surefire way to get them to go to sleep. This surefire way may not be 100 percent surefire, but I'm sharing it with you anyway. Sit back comfortably on a chair or a couch. Put your elbow at a 90-degree angle with your palm facing up and your forearm resting comfortably on your thigh. Gently lie the baby on their back with their head resting in the palm of your hand. Their body will naturally fit into your forearm area. Cross their arms with your other hand. Then begin to slowly bounce your leg up and down. This is my patented sleep strategy.

A few more miscellaneous tips:

- For the first few weeks when the doctors want you to track pee and poop diapers, they sometimes give you a paper journal. Just download an app that allows multiple people to add info. It's so much easier. And when you're delirious and can't remember the last time the baby ate or pooped, it will come in handy.

- Envelope necklines on baby onesies mean that when there is a poop blowout (and there *will* be poop blowouts), you can slide the baby up and out through neckline, allowing the dirty onesie to be pulled down the baby's hips (and preventing poop from getting on their torso or head).

- Zippered pajamas are the way to go. No one has time to deal with a zillion snaps when changing a newborn's many diapers.

- White noise machines are great for helping babies sleep longer. The sound masks all kinds of noises so you can watch TV, have a normal conversation, or do dishes without accidentally waking them.

- Overtired newborns won't sleep. Research "sleep begets sleep" and thank us later.

Just as we have shared these tips with you from our experience, you will also have things that you will experience, strategies you develop, and little nuances about your baby that are unexplainable to everyone else but very natural to you. When it comes to your baby, *you* will be the expert and the go-to for everything. That's exciting. And that's the thing to keep in the forefront of your mind: You have this awesome opportunity to start from ground zero. To build, teach, and create history with your family. We believe it is a dream come true to have a blank canvas and the chance to build from the ground up.

Big-Picture Reminders for Tough Nights

Inevitably, there will be times when the postpartum period feels harder than usual. The following points are meant to encourage you when you're feeling frustrated, stuck, or overwhelmed. If you and/or your partner are struggling and nothing seems to help, then talk to your healthcare provider. They may have other ways to support you.

PROGRESS, NOT PERFECTION. Parenting a newborn is hard. It's an understandable adjustment period. To go from caring for yourself to being up at 3:00 a.m., deliriously trying to calm and feed a newborn who you just met will take some time. Try to be intentional about identifying the progress you make and not focus so much on doing everything perfectly. Your goal is progress, not perfection. Does this week feel even a tiny bit easier than last week? Then you're doing great and on the right path.

IT GETS EASIER. There is a saying that new parents often hear: "The days are long, but the years are short." In the thick of postpartum life, it's easy to forget that what you're experiencing that night, week, or month is temporary. But as the baby grows—as you grow—the day-to-day experience of raising a newborn will get easier. For many new parents, the six-week mark is when postpartum life starts to feel ... doable. By this point, a rough routine has started to form, the baby is a little more social (maybe even smiling!), and parents may feel a smidge more confident.

TINY VICTORIES MATTER. When you're feeling overwhelmed, it helps to focus on what's immediately in front of you, within your control. Look for what's not going wrong and live in that moment as best you can. There may be more to feel okay about than you initially realize. Intentionally celebrate these achievements, no matter how small or insignificant they might seem. You took a shower today? Woo-hoo! The baby fell asleep in the stroller while you were taking a walk? High five! Celebrating these moments will remind you that you're making progress and thus doing a good job. Tiny victories become large victories.

YOUR INTUITION IS WISE. This magical thing happens when we have children: We naturally start to understand some things that we cannot explain to others. Just like you can sense with your partner, you'll know when your kids are uncomfortable, in a bad mood, or extremely excited about something. You'll know when something's not right and when things are just right. Use your intuitive knowledge of your family's needs to help you make decisions, especially when the answers are not always clear. Pause, check in with yourself, and try to sense what your gut is telling you. You may be pleasantly surprised by what happens.

The love you have for your family will lead you in the correct direction, and no amount of knowledge or absorption of content can replace your inner wisdom and instincts. This is your family, and you know them best. Take care of one another, operate from a place of love and peace, and enjoy this new stage of your life. Some of life's best moments await you.

DIVIDE AND CONQUER

You have the rest of your lives to divide and conquer as you raise the latest addition to your family. Be sure to lean into your strengths and divide the parenting and household responsibilities in the ways that feel most comfortable and most equal to you. Remember this does not mean even fifty-fifty splits in every area.

TIME-SENSITIVE

- Schedule newborn checkups
- Schedule lactation consultant
- Schedule postpartum checkups
- Obtain birth certificate and social security card
- Add baby to insurance plan

SCHEDULE AND PLAN

- Survival sleep schedules for *both* parents
- Any spiritual or cultural ceremonies
- Newborn photos
- Date night
- Family outing
- Couple check-in

RESEARCH AND DISCUSS

- Baby formula
  - Premade versus powder
  - Bottles and nipples
- Baby sleep
  - Safe sleep guidelines
  - Naps and wake windows
- Baby digestion
  - Gas, burping, farting
- Postpartum depression

ADDITIONAL

RESOURCES

WEEKS 23–27: REGISTRY, BABYMOON, AND PEDIATRICIANS

Gestational Diabetes Test (page 91)

Catherine Donaldson-Evans, "What to Eat Before the Glucose Test for Best
Results," What to Expect, September 17, 2021, whattoexpect.com/wom/
pregnancy/3-secret-ways-to-pass-the-glucose-test-your-doctor-may-
not-tell-you-about.aspx

WEEKS 32–35: NESTING AND DOCUMENTING

Documenting (page 123)

Mama Bump Rentals: mamabumprentals.com

WEEKS 36–40: LAST-MINUTE PREPARATIONS

Advocate, Advocate, Advocate (page 125)

4Kira4Moms: 4kira4moms.com

CHILDBIRTH: LABOR AND DELIVERY

Team Toolbox (page 142)

Contraction Apps: Full Term—Contraction Timer; Contraction
Timer & Counter 9m

Baby Feeding (page 163)

Bumble Baby: bumblebabychicago.com

Postpartum Depression (page 159)

Postpartum Support International: postpartum.net; hotline 1-800-944-4773

Mayo Clinic, "Postpartum Depression," mayoclinic.org/diseases-conditions/ postpartum-depression/symptoms-causes/syc-20376617

Georgetown University School of Nursing, "Postpartum Depression: Signs and Resources for Help," June 25, 2019, online.nursing.georgetown.edu/ blog/postpartum-depression-resources

REFERENCES

American College of Obstetricians and Gynecologists. "FAQs: Prenatal Genetic Screening Tests," acog.org/womens-health/faqs/prenatal-genetic-screening-tests.

Cleveland Clinic, "Fetal Development: Stages of Growth," my.clevelandclinic .org/health/articles/7247-fetal-development-stages-of-growth.

Cleveland Clinic, "Midwife," my.clevelandclinic.org/health/articles/22648-midwife.

Cleveland Clinic, "Pregnancy: Ovulating, Conception & Getting Pregnant," my.clevelandclinic.org/health/articles/11585-pregnancy-ovulation-conception--getting-pregnant.

Jamila Taylor, Anna Bernstein, Thomas Waldrop, and Vina Smith-Ramakrishnan, "The Worsening U.S. Maternal Health Crisis in Three Graphs," Century Foundation, March 2, 2022, tcf.org/content/commentary/worsening-u-s-maternal-health-crisis-three-graphs/?agreed=1.

Kenneth J. Gruber, Susan H. Cupito, and Christina F. Dobson, "Impact of Doulas on Healthy Birth Outcomes," *Journal of Perinatal Education* 22, no. 1 (Winter 2013): 49–58. doi: 10.1891/1058-1243.22.1.49.

Mayo Clinic, "First Trimester Screening," mayoclinic.org/tests-procedures/first-trimester-screening/about/pac-20394169.

Mayo Clinic, "Labor and Delivery, Postpartum Care," mayoclinic.org/healthy-lifestyle/labor-and-delivery/in-depth/stages-of-labor/art-20046545.

U.S. Equal Employment Opportunity Commission, "Pregnancy Discrimination," eeoc.gov/pregnancy-discrimination.

World Population Review, "Child Care Costs by State 2022," worldpopulationreview.com/state-rankings/child-care-costs-by-state.

INDEX

ACKNOWLEDGMENTS

First, we have to acknowledge Taj and Aaliyah. Beyond the obvious of not being able to write this book without them being here, they are a joy to raise. The experience of parenting them has taught us more about ourselves than we could have ever imagined, and for that we are thankful.

We would not be here today if it weren't for the amazing love, support, and contributions of our family and friends. Raising children is a series of trial and error, and the saying "It takes a village to raise a child" could not be more true. Whether being physically involved or just sharing experiences, we are thankful for all those who have given their time in the support of our children and our journey as parents. Special thanks to the Brown family and Jelks family for contributing their personal experiences to help enrich this book.

ABOUT THE AUTHORS

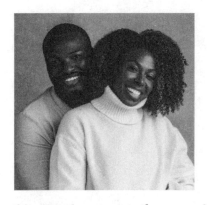

D'ANTHONY WARD is a social media influencer, YouTuber, filmmaker, and the owner of the inspirational clothing brand Create Dope Humans. D'Anthony has worked to disrupt FOMO culture by encouraging his audience to slow down, celebrate the simple things, and appreciate the every day. He is committed to tackling outdated stereotypes around fatherhood, marriage, and parenting. Visit him at thedadvlog.com, on Instagram @dad_vlog, and at createdopehumans.com.

RACHEL WARD helps young people define and achieve their career goals through program development, mentoring, and coaching. She guides young, diverse leaders to showcase their talents and break into challenging industries where they have been historically underrepresented. She also serves on the board of directors of educational STEM nonprofits and passionately identifies ways to advocate for the next generation. As a career-driven mom, Rachel actively promotes a healthy work-life balance. Follow her on Instagram @heyrachelward.

D'Anthony and Rachel live in Atlanta with their two children, Taj and Aaliyah. This is the couple's first book together.

NOTES

NOTES

NOTES

NOTES

NOTES

Hi there,

We hope you enjoyed *The Couples' Pregnancy Guide*. If you have any questions or concerns about your book, or have received a damaged copy, please contact customerservice@penguinrandomhouse.com. We're here and happy to help.

Also, please consider writing a review on your favorite retailer's website to let others know what you thought of the book!

Sincerely,
The Zeitgeist Team